Undo Diabetes
Heal Heart
Lose Weight

A Story of Trial and Transformation

COURAGE – COMMITMENT – COMPLIANCE

Arjit Mahal

Foreword by Dr. Pardeep Aujla

Preface by Dr. Jatinder Aujla

Technics Publications

TECHNICS PUBLICATIONS

TECHNOLOGY / LEADERSHIP

2 Lindsley Road, Basking Ridge, NJ 07920 USA
https://www.TechnicsPub.com

Edited by Susan Toth
Cover design by Lorena Molinari
Images by Lindsay Hopkins

First Printing 2021
Copyright © 2021 by Arjit Mahal

ISBN, print ed.	9781634629379
ISBN, Kindle ed.	9781634629386
ISBN, ePub ed.	9781634629393
ISBN, PDF ed.	9781634629409

Library of Congress Control Number: 2021939476

This book is dedicated to Millie, my loving wife, partner, friend, and well-wisher of half a century. I am grateful for her dedication to my lifestyle, my career, and to the life challenges and triumphs, she has willingly shared with me.

For her support in my health and wellness, this book is an expression of my immense gratitude.

In Millie's name, I gift this to humanity.

Arjit Mahal has written an outstanding book of the utilization of the Dean Ornish diet and wellness program among other health protocols in the treatment of: Type 2 Diabetes Mellitus, Type 1.5 Diabetes Mellitus, Coronary Heart Disease, Obesity, Hypertension, and Hyperlipidemia

This book should be in the hands of all medical students and available in all the medical schools.

The individual who follows the protocol of this book, has information available which can potentially save thousands of lives.

The dietary approach is in the first order of treatments; medications, surgeries etc. should be secondary.

I highly recommend this book.

Dr. Francis J. Cinelli, D.O.

Pennsylvania, USA

April 2021

Contents

Acknowledgments

In my quest for better health, I am indebted to many people during my lifetime. However, it is my health transformation in recent years, which inspired me to write this book. I express my gratitude to the following.

Millie Mahal: My wife of fifty years has endured many hardships related to my health and healing. She has sacrificed in many ways to help me adapt to my new approach to diet by coaching me in the basics of cooking while putting up with my idiosyncrasies. I am grateful for her unselfish devotion to my life and living. This book would not have been possible without her inspiration (even though she did not know I was writing it; it was a surprise gift to her on our 50th marriage anniversary).

Captain Hardarshan Singh Paul: We have been friends for about fifty years. His quest for a spiritual path and our exchange of ideas about health and reversing diabetes has been immensely valuable. I have been a fortunate beneficiary of his research and wisdom.

Family Members: Harpreet Dhillon: for introducing me to InstantPot and answering many of my questions about Indian food ingredients. Jagjot Nagra: for introducing me to the idea of ancient grains and ancient Indian wisdom on food and health. Apara Mahal Sylvester, my daughter, for providing me with resources for book editing and graphics. I am very thankful to all.

Physicians: Dr. Howard Noveck for taking care of my heart for over 30 years. Dr. Sharan Mahal and Dr. Lakhjit Sandhu: They have always been there for me when I needed a second opinion or simply needed comforting assurances. Dr. Harnish Chawla: for enrolling me in the Ornish Lifestyle Medicine program, a game-changer. Dr. Francis Cinelli: When others said not much could be done about an autoimmune problem, he said let us find a solution. Dr. Ramaya Vedula, my endocrinologist, for her state of the art practice, advice, and for introducing me to the CGM tool. Dr. Carl Ingrassia for his excellent podiatric care. Nurse Practitioner Mary Stein has been extremely helpful in my heart therapy program over the years; her compassion and care are unmatched. To all the above, I am indebted for your support.

Hunterdon Cardiopulmonary Rehabilitation, Hunterdon Healthcare, Flemington, New Jersey. Under the superb leadership of Lisa Buckley and Christine Tucker, the entire Ornish Lifestyle Medicine Program Team provided me and others with competent training and coaching, which made a big difference in my health transformation journey. I am indebted to this "Dream Team" of professionals. (Also, my thanks to the Ornish cohorts for their comradery in training).

My extreme gratitude to Dr. Pardeep Aujla and Dr. Jatinder Aujla for reading the manuscript and providing valuable input regarding medical information, and sharing their practical and profound insights. Dr. P. Aujla had in the past shared with me her own experience with treating diabetes and experimenting with fasting herself. I had paid attention to her wisdom. Dr. J. Aujla took time to improve on several medical statements to ensure that the readers would easily understand and "get it."

The Editor: Susan Toth has provided superb editing in correcting my shortcomings in punctuation, grammar, and formatting. I am confident that her slogan will become a reality: *"I'll make your book the one they can't put down!"*

The Publisher: Steve Hoberman of Technics Publications, for many years, has been a colleague, a friend, and publisher of some of my books. It is through his encouragement that after my first book, I continued to write more. After the hard work of finishing my first book, I made a comment to him that I am done writing. He smiled and said, "You will write another book and then another…it is addictive." You are right, Steve. I express my gratitude to Mr. Hoberman and his competent staff for supporting my book.

Foreword

As a primary care provider, I do enjoy the educated consumer. I see Mr. Mahal's dilemma with his diabetes. From my end, there's also frustration when I have a patient who does not care or take any part in their care. I have been practicing for over 18 years. As physicians, we often deal with diseases that have no cure, no rationale, and may have bleak outcomes. I always find ways to simplify the treatment plan for a patient, so there is more compliance for a desirable outcome.

It is very rewarding to see a good report on a follow-up session. I have noticed that patients who leave everything to the physician generally never have good results. I remind them often that the physician is just a guide who helps the patient identify the problem, determine an accurate diagnosis, and lay out the best plan to solve the problem. If a physician is the GPS (Global Positioning System), the patient is the driver who must have a vested interest in reaching the desired destination.

Most people accept the diagnosis as the normal aging process or blame it on their family history. Some question "why me?" Very few ask the most important question, how can I undo this or what do I need to do to reverse this?"

It is a dream of a physician to have a patient come to the office fully prepared with questions, progress notes, home readings, labs, etc., done. This collaborative approach reduces my time reviewing, questioning, and closing off that dead space that can be used for tackling the actual problem. When efforts fail, new plans can be made. However, when no attempt is made on the part of the patient, then there is not much to add except more pills.

Arjit Mahal always inspired me with his dedication to reversing his diabetes, I enjoy discussing his medical roadmap with him and often learn more myself. I often use some of his knowledge to educate my patients. His understanding of the physiology behind his medical conditions is very impressive. He struggled to lose weight until he found multiple resources and recommendations to improve his health. If one strategy didn't work, he tried another. He showed that nothing is impossible.

While most people sat at home during the COVID-19 pandemic and complained about the situation, Mr. Mahal not only fulfilled his goal but worked on this book to help others like him.

This book is like an already prepared meal; all you have to do is eat.

Pardeep Aujla, MD
Massachusetts, USA
February 2021

Preface

With full disclosure, I have known Arjit Mahal for over 43 years. He is a mentor, a friend, and a wealth of knowledge. I would say what strikes me the most about him is his reluctance to the status quo. As I am a physician, he would bounce things off me from time to time. Regarding his diabetes, I would simply tell him, "lose weight." I should have told him "win the lottery" and see if his due diligence could have figured that out!

I witnessed his meticulous notetaking and asking questions that patients often are too embarrassed to broach. But as with most things, he persevered and didn't just think outside the box; he figured out the composition of the box. As I read through this book, I found myself looking back at old medical school textbooks to figure out what he was talking about. Arjit has distilled the essence of diabetes and the factors that lead to the vicious cycle of this unrelenting disease.

If you've picked up this book and thumbed through the pages, you'll see diagrams, quotes, charts, and all manner of data. If that's too much for you, thank Arjit for the painstaking hours he spent trying to help others like him. You may not understand all of it, but you'll be better off for the effort. You see, Mr. Mahal learned long ago that you shouldn't just take what's fed to you. If he did, he would be on more insulin, probably over 200 pounds having some doctors tell him "lose weight, and that lottery thing too."

Besides learning about his condition and how to fight it without adding to his medical copay, he researched and learned to sacrifice. As a physician, I can tell you that there's always more pills to add to a regimen. But what about those patients who want to roll back the years and not just keep putting Band-Aids on things? Well, you're in luck; this book is an excellent start. Unfortunately, a sizable population sees diabetes as a permanent condition. But as Arjit has detailed, you can put up a fight, and if your will is strong, you come out the other end better off.

I often tell patients when they ask for medication that I have the best pill. As they sit there, I tell them "personal responsibility." They usually don't like that. As you read through Arjit's diet, you'll see what I mean. Sure, everyone wants a cheeseburger, steak, fried chicken, but at what cost?

If you've come to this place, you'll be assured that you're not alone. Take what he offers, polish it up, add/subtract/divide, but get involved. As one of my favorite bands once said, "Life is not a rehearsal."

Jatinder Aujla, MD
Massachusetts, USA, February 2021

Disclaimer

This book is a narrative of the author's personal experience and success in reversing his diabetes, improving his heart health, and losing weight with an overall enhancement of his general well-being.

To understand and address how the complexities of his medical challenges, and the knowledge of technical considerations he has gained during this experience, are interpreted and expressed in this book are for his own use only. This includes health, nutrition, diet, fasting, fitness, stress management, and general well-being. The techniques, strategies, and suggestions expressed here are intended for awareness only.

The contents of this book are NOT intended as medical diagnosis, solution, or treatment; the book is NOT a substitute for medical advice. This book is also NOT intended as advice on nutrition, foods, and supplements in general. The data, information, concepts, tool, templates, and techniques in the text are shown by the author by how he manages his health goals.

The reader must consult appropriate and qualified medical practitioners, nutritionists, and experts in other relevant disciplines before using any of the ideas and opinions expressed by the author. These may not be approved by FDA.

While the author has made every effort to provide accurate telephone numbers, internet addresses, and other contact information at the time of publication, neither the publisher nor the author assumes any responsibility for errors or changes after publication. Further, the publisher does not have any control over and does not assume any responsibility for the author or third-party websites or their content.

Neither the publisher nor the author is engaged in rendering professional advice or services to the individual reader. The ideas, procedures, and suggestions contained in this book are not intended as a substitute for consulting with your physician. All matters regarding your health require medical supervision. Neither the author nor the publisher shall be liable or responsible for any loss or damage allegedly arising from any information or suggestion in this book.

Declaration: The Author has no vested interest, financial or otherwise, in any of the products and services mentioned in this book. He has no personal interest in promoting any individual, any business entity, brand, or a specific doctrine — whatsoever.

About the Book

Health is worth more than learning.

Thomas Jefferson

Authors of some books write because their subconscious tells them to write. They have no option but to transfer their know-how onto paper—to give rest to their impatient, innovative mind. There is serendipity manifested in the pieces of the puzzle when a story comes together in such an initiative. The author, then, is only a facilitator of words and sentences. This is such a book.

To understand my two health issues, diabetes and chronic heart disease, I had read many books over the years and consulted with my physicians for solutions to make sense of it all. My dog-eared book pages, with highlighted passages and paper notes, were all over the place. When I needed to reference a topic, I had to search the location of the topics in various books repeatedly. I had decided to consolidate my notes in one single source, a Word document. After typing up several pages of disparate but related information, I realized there was a book in the making. The result is what you are reading now.

I am not a physician, scientist, or nutritionist, nor do I have any vested interest to support any solution offered by any business entity for their products and services. I have simply written this book for my personal reference and for sharing with others for awareness. By writing, one gets a deeper understanding of a subject and one's own self.

I am a published author and had a successful career in the corporate world, followed by the founding of a profitable consulting organization. In my professional retirement, I am not looking to make money by selling this book and open an account in a Swiss bank, so to say. This is a not-for-profit book. Any royalty I will receive from the sale of my books will support charities that support nature, humans, and animals.

This book is a labor of love with the following mission:

By "reversing" my diabetes and attempting to "reverse" my heart disease, with the positive achievement of weight reduction and general well-being, I have gained knowledge and experience which I want to share with others—for awareness and inspiration."

My principle of writing: **"Write with your heart and write for yourself!"**

This means that I am writing with sincerity, all that I know currently to the best of my ability. And I am writing for my personal satisfaction, in that if anyone picked my book and gained something out of it—I would have contributed to humanity. I had spent many years in the Learning and Development practice of implementing a *Learning Framework* in a large organization worldwide. This framework was inspired by the research of the *Center for Creative Leadership* over several decades. This proven concept, irrespective of any disciple or field, states people learn by 70/20/10 approach. They learn 10% from formal training and reading books, 20% from others such as coaches, mentors, and colleagues, and 70% by doing. In the topic of self-health improvement, the content of this book, I have practiced this framework—and I believe; therefore, that qualifies me for my contribution to society.

Since the topics cover medical and scientific thinking, I refer to valid sources, paraphrase, and summarize issues as I understand them, both in text and conceptual diagrams. I suggest readers go deeper into these topics for their own interpretations.

I am a 73-year-old male, a Punjabi Sikh, from Punjab, India, who migrated to America some 52 years ago. I have two chronic medical conditions: Diabetes type 2 (Later diagnosed as type 1.5 called LADA, *Latent Autoimmune Diabetes in Adults,* and have CHD, Coronary Heart

Disease.) I am an active and productive individual with a positive attitude toward life and living.

As a diabetic patient, I was on one medication, then two, and so on, until the doctor put me on insulin a couple of years ago. Herein lies the first problem: if something does not work, a different approach is warranted. Medications should be added and withdrawn with the same scrutiny. My weight started to increase, just about one pound a month with no stopping in sight, no matter what diet I tried or how much exercise I did. I used to be about 170 pounds; it went up to over 190 pounds. In a perfect world, I would weigh about 150 to 155 pounds. Our body, as complex as it is, is hard-wired to function at its optimal weight. The more weight you gain, the resources of your body try to accommodate, but they do have a limit. Conversely, your waist gets bigger, and your wallet soon must also make the same sacrifice. With each passing month, the four-times-a-day insulin intake had to be increased gradually. That is when I realized that the more insulin I took, the more my weight would go up. The more my weight went up, the more insulin I needed.

Health service providers never mentioned to me that there could be alternate approaches such as managing diabetes with diet and fasting, as an example. After reading two books on reversing diabetes through a plant-based diet and fasting regimen, I decided to try on my own. Being mostly vegetarian, I found it somewhat easier to start on my own, but fasting was a challenge. I had many questions about this topic for which my doctors were not any help, and I could not reach those physician authors whose books I had read. I went ahead on my own—my solo journey.

On the heart side, I had a different situation. One area of the heart where one artery bifurcates into two had a blockage which was fixed with stent implants. Two and three years later, the same arteries had blockages again. My cardiologist enrolled me in a nine-week Dean Ornish reversing heart disease program called *Ornish Lifestyle Medicine,* which includes four interrelated parts: nutrition, fitness, stress management, and love and support. It was offered by the Cardiac Rehab Department of my local hospital. This was a game-changer for me. Combined with my own effort already underway, this program and the guidance provided by the Rehab Staff gave me many tools to continue my plant-based diet (and fasting on my own). My progress was closely monitored, and periodically my reports were sent to my cardiologist for his review.

"Hypertension, Diabetes, and CHD are partners in crime. Understand diabetes is like a flame thrower to your vessels, and nothing is spared."

I read books of the doctors who promoted plant-based solutions and participated in the reversing heart ideas program. In addition, I read several other books on fasting and nutrition. The result is that I am in a much better place in terms of management of my heart disease, diabetes, and body weight.

This book is not an academic or a scientific paper, nor does it have any case studies. I have included a few simple recipes which I had learned to suit my new diet regimen. Consider these to be starter templates to experiment with—and then improvise as needed. In layman's terms, it is my personal story of health and healing through self-research and self-determination.

The scope of the book includes my experience with the healing journey of the following:

- Diabetes type 2 and type 1.5 (LADA). (type 1.5 diabetes is in some way like type 1 diabetes, but I have not self-studied that condition, and therefore it is **NOT** in the scope.)

- Cardiac Heart Disease (CHD) in terms of Atherosclerosis prevention is within my purview (other heart-related issues are **NOT** in scope).

- Weight Management: The outcome of resulting plant-based diet and fasting. Other numerous diet methods such as low carbs, all fat, and calorie counting, are **NOT** in the scope because I have never used those methods and don't have an interest in counting calories, carbs, and such.

As I am not a medical professional, I had to read and re-read the books and articles to understand the complexities of the anatomy and body's processes that interplay with diseases. To understand the technicalities, I drew my own diagrams, made my own notes, and tried my best to understand the intricacies of the biological processes. Therefore, in this book, I am keeping the language simple to express my knowledge and experience gained—in my own simple way. (Those who are looking for detailed technical data, this book is not for them).

Albert Einstein had once stated: *Everything should be made as simple as possible, but no simpler.* Simpler would mean diluting the intended meaning of the topic at hand. Conversely, I am not qualified to go into technical details and don't pretend that I know what I don't know. Therefore, I had to keep a balance between the simple and the simpler. The medical professionals reading this book may take exception to my simplified narratives and graphics and description of the medical concepts—as I best understand. They must note that this book is written from the lens of a consumer, me, the patient. The lens of the practitioners would be obviously more technical. I invite them to read this book from a patient's point of view before making any judgment. There may be takeaways that would enhance their own professional development (remember the 20% of the learning framework: learning from others).

Chapter Summaries

- **Know Thyself**: In this chapter, the emphasis is made on taking charge of your body's health-related considerations to ensure that you are the master of your own destiny. Some principles are provided to help in self-transformation: Courage, Commitment, and Compliance.

- **Self-Advocacy:** Some people in medical science, research scientists, and the pharma industry have their own agendas, which many times keep the consumer in the dark or mislead them. So, how do we make sense of the mass of information that comes at us from all directions? Here I have outlined some principles that helped me become a better consumer—for my own good.

- **Digestive System:** Digestion is one of the critical functions our body must perform to survive and thrive. The food we eat provides necessary nutrients that supply our cells with sustenance and energy. This chapter sets a baseline of the body's food intake and digestion process, facilitating the understanding of the chapter on diabetes.

- **Diabetes:** In this chapter, I describe the genesis of my diabetes condition, the progressive state of increased medications, my experience with what I could or could not learn from the medical practitioners, and medical science. The hope came to me by some books—which put me on a track to success.

- **The Heart:** My primary condition has been Coronary Heart Disease (CHD). So, the focus of reversing heart disease is based on my condition and practice of a methodology—that has worked for me: Ornish Lifestyle Medicine.

- **Weight:** Certain medications for diabetes caused my weight to increase. By understanding the insulin resistance mechanism, I learned that it is a vicious cycle of insulin-weight gain-more inulin-more weight gain. I share my achievement in this regard.

- **Nutrition:** This is where I go into the detail of my own food practices based on a plant-based diet. I discuss some issues and considerations for self-managing one's own eating practice by establishing good food and good eating principles.

- **Fasting:** Based on the process of Autophagy, I explain in simple terms how I started the fasting program and managed it successfully. For ages, many cultures have been fasting. It is not easy but doable and pays good dividends in better healing and health.

- **Tools:** This outlines my "arsenal" of techniques, devices, and templates, which helped me establish my goals for healing and maintaining good health.

- **Conclusion:** In this chapter, I share my latest health data after having been able to maintain and sustain my goals of diabetes management, heart-healing, weight management, and general well-being.

- **References:** Most of the sources of material used in this book are outlined in this section. This includes books, periodicals, and websites.

All the good in this book is through the blessing of my ancestors; any faulty deductions or omissions are to be ascribed to me.

"I shall pass this way but once; any good that I can do or any kindness I can show to any human being; let me do it now. Let me not defer nor neglect it, for I shall not pass this way again." ~ Etienne De Grellet, French Quaker Missionary

---

Acronyms

This section has a glossary of acronyms mentioned several times in the book. The definitions of the medical, scientific, and nutritional terms can be extraordinarily complex, and experts are needed in individual disciplines to decipher those. The acronyms used in this book are limited to the mission and scope of the content.

A1c	hemoglobin A1C or HbA1c	**GI**	Glycemic Index
AD	Alzheimer's disease	**GP**	General Practitioner
AGP	Ambulatory Glucose Profile Report	**Hs-CRP**	high-sensitivity C-reactive protein (hs-CRP) test,
BMI	Body Mass Index	**HDL**	High-Density Lipoprotein
eAg	Estimated Average Glucose	**IF**	Intermittent Fasting
CABG	Coronary Artery Bypass Grafting	**LAD**	Left Anterior Descending Artery
CAD	Coronary Artery Disease	**LADA**	Latent Autoimmune Diabetes in Adults
CDSR	Cohrane Database of Systematic Review	**LDL**	Low-Density Lipoprotein

CGM	Continuous Glucose Monitor	**LIMA**	Left Internal Mammary Artery
CDC	Center for Disease Control & Prevention	**METS**	Metabolic Equivalence. Physiological Measurement
CHD	Chronic Heart Disease	**MFMER**	Mayo Foundation for Medical Education and Research
CPIR	Cephalic Phased Insulin Release	**SMART**	Specific, Measurable, Achievable, Relevant, Timebound
CVD	Cardiovascular Disease	**TCA**	Tricarboxylic
DNA	Deoxyribonucleic Acid	**TIR**	Time in Range
FDA	Food Drug Administration	**WHO**	World Health Organization
FF	Flexible Fasting	**WHR**	Waist Hip Ratio
GMI	Glucose Management Indicator		

CHAPTER 1

Know Thyself

All human actions have one or more of these seven causes:
chance, nature, compulsion, habit, reason, passion, and desire.
Aristotle (384 BC-322 BC)

Humans are biological organisms and part of the animal kingdom. We have our own unique intelligence type, while all living organisms have their own type for their own survival. Sigmund Freud, the Austrian neurologist, best known for developing the theories and techniques of psychoanalysis, had suggested that the purpose of life is survival and pursuit of happiness. How do we feel that happiness? Perhaps in our "minds"? Where does the "mind" reside in our body? And what is its role? Could it be to think and influence our decisions? It has been said that biology gave us a brain, we created the mind. Is this our own creation that enables us to survive and thrive? I leave this question for the philosophers and the scientists to figure out.

However, we need to "think" about ourselves first and foremost. (In "spiritual" terms, if I don't exist, my world does not exist, and this universe does not exist.) But if I can sense that I AM, then for that moment, I do exist.

Who am I?

This most important question for an individual human being should be Who Am I? One should post a sticky note on the bathroom mirror with this statement and look at this question every morning.

Human beings are a "microcosm, a condensation of the entire · universe."

Paracelsus 1493-1541

We are merely an organism that came biologically into existence and one day will die. The space in between birth and death is what we call LIFE. It is merely a minute event in the history of the universe—irrespective of our social status, wealth, or social strata. Except that we have created a concept of "mind." We are animals, and I wonder if the animals know they have a mind?

We have a body, a biologically fine-tuned machine provided by nature. We can call nature "God" or give it any other name if you like. I don't want to comment on the topic of religious dogmas, doctrines, or beliefs associated with it. Beliefs may not always be true, in my opinion. On the earth, we believe the sun rises in the East, but we can't say that if we are sitting in a space station many miles above the earth. Beliefs are merely beliefs! Then what is the truth?

Many messiahs have come and gone. Their disciples have perpetuated their philosophy on the masses for ages. No one has been able to describe the Truth—the absolute Truth because they themselves were possibly on the quest to know the unknown, and maybe they could only perceive what might be. The idea that some divine providence would take care of our life is possibly a hope. Hope is never a strategy. Then each of us is on our own to survive and thrive, the best we can be with what we have till it lasts. In the Indian philosophy, it is said, *"Himate marda, madde khuda"* (God helps those who help themselves).

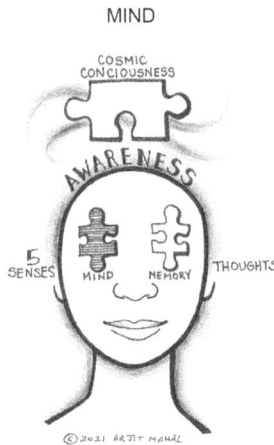

Figure 1.1 Mind, Sub-Conscious

Mind

In the human brain, MIND, invoked by lifelong experiences through the stimulus of all human senses, is a repository of memories and perceptive knowledge—of one's own universe. (Every individual has his/her own "perceptive universe".)

Mind is the "energy" that invokes a continuous stream of wandering THOUGHTS that may result in actions; The ACTIONS may be positive or negative and may sometimes result in unintended outcomes.

Through THOUGHTS, the MIND manifests moment-to-moment with continuous change in sense impressions and mental phenomena. The MIND must be "watched" closely to ensure that it may not lead one's desired intent astray—often overriding the "divine" wisdom offered by the SUB-CONSCIOUS. (The purpose of meditation is to purge such thoughts and bring peace to the mind.)

"When the mind is calm and centered, it can turn inward. Only a mind turned inward can experience the vastness and beauty of the Divine Consciousness…When the river is calm, the reflection is clearer. When the mind is calm, there is greater clarity in the field of expression. Our sense of observation, perception, and expression improve. As a result, we are able to communicate effectively and clearly."
~ *The Secret of Mantra Chanting*, By Ravi Shankar.

Man Jeeta; Jagjeet. (To win over one's mind is to win the world!)

Guru Nanak

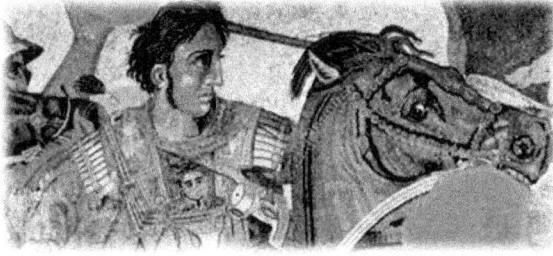

Figure 1.2 Alexander in India

Alexander the Great, Alexander III of Macedon, commonly known as Alexander the Great, was a king of the ancient Greek kingdom. In Asia, he was known as *Sikander*. After conquering Asia Minor, Persia, and other empires on the way, he arrived in India in 326 BC. He camped on the bank of river Indus before the Battle of Hydaspes (now Jelum River). Sikander was fond of talking to holy persons. Sitting on the bank of the river was a Sadhu, an ascetic, with hardly any clothes on—sitting in meditation. Sikander asked his aids to bring this sadhu to him for conversation. When the aid asked the sadhu to come and meet Sikander, the sadhu refused. He was reminded by the aid that Sikander-a-Azam, the conqueror of the world, is inviting him to meet him, and he dared to refuse? "I don't know any *Sikander Shikander*. If he wants to meet me, he can come here," said the sadhu defiantly.

On hearing this, Sikander got off his horse and went to meet the sadhu. "Sit by me and tell me what you are doing here?" said the sadhu. "I am Sikander-a-Azam. In ten years, I have conquered half of the world; now I have conquered India," said Sikander. Sadhu further asked, "What are you going to do next?"

Sikander: I am on my way to conquer the rest of the world.

Sadhu: Then what are you going to do?

Sikander: I will go to my home in Greece and rest in peace.

Sadhu: Causing all the mayhem and suffering, if you are just looking for peace, come sit by me, and meditate. You will find the peace right here—within yourself.

On his next march toward river Hyphasis (now Beas River), it is said that his army was about to mutiny. He had decided to return West and set sail on the Indus River. Maybe Sikander had heeded the sadhu's wisdom. It's all in the mind!

Take Charge

You don't have to be a physician to know the functioning of your own body. Read, research, and be knowledgeable in human anatomy at a basic level. There are systems created by nature: the digestive system, heart system, skin system, organs and their functions, brain system, and so on. When you get a report of your blood work, study it, understand it, and ask questions of your medical practitioner. File the report so you can compare it in the future to assess any changes. Over the years, I have asked people if they took a copy of their bloodwork report and filed it for future reference. Many times, the answer is no! But if they have their car serviced for an oil change or tire change, they will have a report filed in a folder for future reference. Your body is more sacred than a car!

All this makes you a smarter consumer—for your own benefit. Physicians have limited time to meet you, check your health issues, and address all the concerns. Be an educated and wise consumer. Have a plan to address your health concerns. Make a list so that you don't forget. Prior to a doctor's visit, do your own research and prepare a list of concerns and questions. Ask the physician about the latest research and medical solutions that could benefit you. Keep your questions to the point and direct. If this approach doesn't work for your doctor, then maybe it's time for you to move on.

I use the following format for all my doctor visits:

Patient Name: XYX

Doctor's Name and Date of appointment

Note: Do your own research on the topic of concern prior to meeting a health provider:

1. Describe how you feel and what might have to be addressed.

2. Describe specific concerns you may have.

3. Review bloodwork or any other test results.

4. Review your medications list (and vitamins and supplements if the practitioners are receptive to this idea and are knowledgeable in micronutrients).

5. Ask the caregiver if, instead of taking medication, can lifestyle changes help.

6. Ask the doctor, "Is there anything else you should know which may have been missed?"

7. Agree on the next steps.

You are paying for the service, and it is your body on the line, so to say.

Maintain Records

Those who are fortunate to have few or no health issues may not appreciate this. However, as we get older, we may likely have multiple health concerns, along with their diagnoses and treatments. Maintaining good records, on paper or electronic or both, makes you more organized for your own health care. Medical service providers like this very much when you have all your history easily available when needed; they respect you more and are likely to pay more attention to your well-being. I also keep my medical information with MedicAlert Foundation, a non-profit entity that makes the records available 24/7 in emergencies. Their toll-free phone number is on a tag around my neck on a chain. (www.medicalert.org). Additionally, there may be other such facilities and tools relevant to one's own needs.

Destiny is not a matter of chance; it is a matter of choice. It is not a thing to be waited for; it is a thing to be achieved.
William Jennings Bryan, political leader, and orator

Destiny could be another concept or belief which may be hard to understand! This is called *Kismet*, or providence in the East. In simple terms, it may be the unknown future— of which we may or may not have any control. However, we can assume safe sailing with some storms on the ocean and move on, rowing the oars of hope and courage.

To embark on a personal transformation such as the one this book is about, there is a need for guiding principles for starting the journey and staying on track. I have these principles: **Courage, Commitment, and Compliance.**

My Health Transformation

How reckless is nature in the distribution of her gifts!

P. G. Wodehouse

English American novelist and humorist

Courage

Destiny deals a "hand of cards" to everyone. Some have good, some have not so good, and some don't have to worry about a thing. It is what it is. So, we take what we have and play life's game with the best possible strategy we can formulate. But this must be done by each one of us—no one should expect others to do it for us. The first thing for any strategy is to be clear about the purpose; in health transformation, it would be the **CAUSE**: What, Where, Why, and Why Now?

In my case, the CAUSE was clear. Three intertwined chronic conditions: Diabetes, Coronary Heart Disease, and Weight Gain.

So, in 2019, after reading some books (which are mentioned in the later chapters), the concept of a plant-based-diet had appealed to me. However, there are numerous labels associated with this form of diet that has different meanings for different people: Vegetarian, Vegan, this, that, and the other. Per *Healthline Magazine* (healthline.com), the main types of veganism eating patterns are whole-food, junk food, raw-food, low-fat, raw-food veganism, and so on.

People want to pigeonhole you with prevalent terms—which mean many things to many people. I would rather say that I am on Mother-Earth-Diet; I eat only what grows above and under the ground. Full Stop! I saw clear benefits for my diabetes and weight management. I was told that diabetes cannot be reversed. What I am trying to do is Diet Managed Diabetes. This was the first time I had heard of this term. It did not matter to me what to call it: reversal or in remission. To not engage anyone in the underlying medical/technical considerations, to keep it simple, I decide to title the book with the term UNDO Diabetes. Sacrifice is essential, and spectators may not see the results they desire.

In 2020, my destiny put me in the hands of my cardiologist, Dr. Harnish Chawla, who is part of the Hunterdon Cardiovascular Associates in Flemington, New Jersey. He recommended that I participate in a reversing heart disease program called *Ornish Lifestyle Medicine,* offered under the care of competent professionals in the Hunterdon Medical Center of the same town. I was unsure what this would offer as I had been twice before over the years in two cardiac rehab programs in different hospitals. I was not sure whether to join or not. My inside voice gave me the courage to sign up. This program, in addition to Mother-Earth-Diet (my term), trained me in other tools such as Fitness, Stress Management, and love and support (of cohorts, the peers in this program, family, and friends). The results were a dramatic change in my blood work, well-being, and the resulting feeling of wholesome goodness overall.

Commitment

"Commitment" has many synonyms in the dictionary: a pledge, vow, promise, duty, obligation, or responsibility. Yes, it takes all this to embark on the programs I have mentioned above. No change is easy, and our minds don't like us to attempt a "road less traveled." The only entity in this world that likes change is a "wet baby!" The journey is full of doubts, contradictory advice from experts, tough questions from your loved ones, friends, and colleagues. They sometimes become doctors, scientists, and experts all in one when they hear what you are up to. But it is interesting, the same people possibly never suggested any corrective ideas earlier! If you have the CAUSE, you must believe in your subconscious. It tells you what the right path is, even though we sometimes ignore it. Silence is a great teacher within; listen to it. It has been said it is better to try and fail rather than never try at all.

Compliance

Once you start seeing the positive outcomes, diabetes starts to be "un-done" (my term). The need for medications is reduced or eliminated, the heart indicators of inflammation and arteriosclerosis are stable, your weight goes down incrementally, and you feel good and wholesome. It is time to stay disciplined and comply with all the protocols you have learned, applied, and used successfully. To ensure compliance, one must use measures as indicators that would show progress.

The term SMART is used in the corporate world to track progress. It also applies to any project and can be used to track the progress of your own Cause and its goals.

SMART is an acronym that you can use to guide your goal setting. Its criteria are commonly attributed to Peter Drucker's Management by Objectives concept. The first known use of the term occurs in the November 1981 issue of *Management Review* by George T. Doran. Since then, Professor Robert S. Rubin (Saint Louis University) wrote about SMART in an article for The Society for Industrial and Organizational Psychology. He stated that SMART has come to mean different things to different people. (Reference source: mindtools.com). To make sure your goals are clear and reachable, each one should be:

✓ **S**pecific (simple, sensible, significant).

✓ **M**easurable (meaningful, motivating).

✓ **A**chievable (agreed, attainable).

✓ **R**elevant (reasonable, realistic, resourced, results-based).

✓ **T**ime-bound (time-based, time-limited, timely, time-sensitive).

The definition of this acronym can be modified to one's own need for tracking health-related goals. For example, lower A1c below 7.0 to be in range with my age group's recommended standard by my next blood test scheduled in the next three months.

As I close this chapter, I am sharing a couple of inspirational phrases I recently read in a new book by Denise Castille: *I Don't Want To Die Like This, A Survivor's Guide To Thriving After a Heart Attack*. **Take the cup by the handle**. The author's mother, who prefers to be addressed as Miss Shirley, used to say this whenever she handed her a cup of tea. It meant "to make it happen...do it." And another saying I find equally profound: **"Triumph or Tragedy...you decide the Trajectory."**

Farewell on the journey – with *Courage, Commitment and Compliance.*

CHAPTER 2

Self-Advocacy

I observe the physician with the same diligence as the disease.
John Donne, British poet, satirist, lawyer, and cleric

The human body is a complex system of biological and chemical processes with various systems having symbiotic dependencies. I admire the physicians, scientists, and philosophers who invest years of their lives in learning the art and science of the human body (and animal bodies) so that they can understand problems, conduct diagnoses, and find solutions. It is indeed a noble profession.

I take this opportunity to express my gratitude to all the medical professionals, pharmacists, pharmaceutical scientists, and medical technology inventors (and my medical insurance providers, both corporate and the Government) who have helped me survive and thrive throughout my life's health journey. I've had many surgeries, chronic issues, but I knew that help was a phone call away or an ambulance ride away. Without their help, I would not be around to write this book!

On Medical Practice

My statements about physicians and their healing intent are not to criticize but to highlight some considerations which have prompted me to take charge of my own body and well-being the best I could and enable the medical practitioners to do the best they can. In the current times of complexity of medical science enabled by ever-improving technology, this is no easy task. The physicians are specialists in particular areas of the body, and it is hard to find someone who can holistically examine the body and ascertain a course of action. Sadly, some physicians are driven by greed, not just by their Hippocratic oath. But there is a majority who are dedicated to their profession and provide the best possible competence.

I must say that the GPs (General Practitioners or Internists) come close to this competence. They then, of course, recommend specialists based on their diagnosis. Dr. Pardeep Aujla offers an analogy of her medical profession with that of an architect. Her role as a GP is like that of an architect who lays the design of a building and, through the blueprints, knows how rooms are connected and what utilities are situated where. For maintenance, the troubleshooting of problems and their resolution becomes relatively convenient to address. And when there is a need for specialized work such as plumbing and electricity, the architect can make an appropriate referral to the specialists.

The issue is with insurance-driven corporate entities that manage the practices. In many cases, they have strict measures of time that can be spent on a patient. They must move fast, the nurse must move fast, and on top of that, they must be computer savvy to add the data on computer screens in real-time. It is well known that our "consciousness" cannot be split—it focuses on one task at a time, unlike the hype promoted falsely by the corporate sector that multitasking can be done. Yes, it can be done at the cost of less attention to one individual event or instance of an activity.

I sit with some of my doctors in the examination room, and they hardly make eye contact with me; they are more focused on data input and sending the prescription online to my pharmacy—and moving on to the next patient. While I understand that physicians are measured for "limiting" time with their patients, if they look into the eyes of a patient and observe their responses and body language, they will understand more about their patients—even if it is five minutes of quality attention.

The single biggest problem in communication is the illusion that it has taken place.

George Bernard Shaw, Irish writer

I don't know if medical schools teach listening skills; however, if a medical practitioner would read this book, here is a bonus I am offering: Listening Skills Tool: *The Listening LADDER.*

Epictetus, the Greek sage and philosopher (AD 55-135), stated: "Nature gave us one tongue and two ears so that we could hear twice as much as we speak." While this advice is good for all humans in all roles, the idea that we should be good listeners has a profound meaning for anyone, especially in the role of a coach, mentor, facilitator, or medical healer. The following technique can be easily mastered with practice.

The Listening LADDER:

- Look: At the person speaking to you. Make eye contact to express that you are interested in what the other person has to say.

- Ask: Questions. Ask open-ended follow-up questions to comprehend the meaning of what is being said by the speaker.

- Don't: Interrupt or be interrupted. Ensure that the interruption is only for the clarification of what has been said.

- Don't: Change the subject. You will get an indication to change the topic when the speaker is finished with one thought. Look for cues to transition to another topic.

- **E**mpathize: With the speaker. Demonstrate this by a gesture such as nodding your head so that the speaker gets the message that you are interested in what is being said.

- **R**espond: Verbally and nonverbally. Through body language, such as nodding your head or eye/eyebrow movements, acknowledge that you are just as engaged in the conversation as the speaker is. You can do this without interrupting the speaker by saying, "…I see…" or "…I understand…."

Medical practitioners, as stated earlier, go through many years of formal education, training, and practice. The body needs nutrients: micronutrients like vitamins and minerals and macronutrients like carbohydrates, fats, and proteins. It is my experience that most practitioners have little or no knowledge of the use of supplements containing vitamins and minerals. I guess that other than their training in anatomy, pathology, or pharmacological medicine, very little is taught on this topic. My guess was confirmed when I read the statement of Kenneth Power, MD, in the Forward of Gin Stephens' book *Delay, Don't Deny*: "…It was once a secret that we physicians are not trained in nutrition; we are experts in pathology and pharmacology..." Having said that, there seem to be only two types of doctors who can provide consultation on supplements: naturopaths and the authors of health books. Next time you see your physician, ask if he or she can recommend you any supplements. Either you may get silence or a copout answer: take multivitamin supplements. In any case, one must be careful to balance taking the vitamins and supplements because excessive intake could be harmful with unintended consequences.

I can't help but share my experience on this topic.

For a second opinion on a serious health issue, I go to a teaching hospital's doctors. They are interested in research and innovation and have knowledge of the latest medicinal research and technology. A few years ago, I had developed a skin condition for which I went to see a dermatologist with over 30 years' experience, who is well known and head of the Department of Dermatology in a prestigious teaching hospital in a big city. During one of my follow-up visits, I asked the doctor, "Is there a supplement I can take to help my skin health in general?" With a smirk on his face, he said no. I challenged him further: "Doctor, being that skin is the largest organ of the human body, does it not need micronutrients which may benefit from supplements?" On a subsequent visit, he sarcastically said to me, "By the way, one of my assistant doctors made a list of cocktails for you." I now had a list of three supplements. Coincidentally, I visited my podiatrist in the same month. While he was examining the skin of the feet, I had asked him the same question I had asked the dermatologist. He replied, "skin craves vitamin E." Bravo, I had some guidance. Since then, I have made it a habit of massaging the skin of my legs and feet with Vitamin E oil.

I wonder why medical colleges don't teach students more about nutrition and micronutrients. It is analogous to automobile engineering students being taught all about the automobile engines and mechanics, except superficial training on what makes the machine function, such as air, petrol, gas, engine oil, and brake fluid.

Since my book's focus is recovering from diabetes and heart healing, I want to mention that each of the experts in these areas focuses on their area of concern. An endocrinologist focuses on the endocrine system, and a cardiologist focuses on the cardiac system. Since I have chronic conditions in both these areas, I know there is an "overlap" or symbiotic relationship between the two and, of course, among other body systems. Generally, no physician would ask questions about the other physician's area of care, thus the need for a GP.

Having diabetes for many years, my cardiologist suggested that I ask my endocrinologist to perform a C-Peptide test to determine if my pancreas was producing insulin. That test showed that, indeed, my pancreas was producing insulin, but my insulin autoantibody was making it less effective. With this knowledge, my diagnosis classification was changed from type 2 to type 1.5 (LADA). With that change, I started to think about what I could do regarding the autoantibody onslaught. After my fasting regimen and other protocols mentioned in more detail in this book, my own pancreas started to make more insulin. By no means am I questioning the competence of my health care providers—I am only bringing a message to the reader that you need to become more knowledgeable about your own body and research and ask questions.

I hope my above observations are not taken as an insult by the medical practitioners. Rather, I am offering an opportunity for them to enhance their competence for their professional self-development.

On Medical Research

Consumers like me who try their best to learn from research and periodicals are kept in the dark or rather lead into a dark tunnel of organized deceit. In the later chapters, I go into more detail about my quest to rid myself of diabetes and keep my heart healthy. Here is one example.

When I decided to focus on plant-based food, I stumbled upon the following article by Dr. Joel Kahn, MD; Posted by The Plant-Based Solution on September 16, 2020 (https://bit.ly/3xahxd4).

The observation that diet and health are related can be traced back at least to Hippocrates over 2,000 years ago with the statement credited to him that "food is medicine". The average lifespan in the last century has been extended greatly, but many of those additional years are burdened with chronic diseases and disabilities. Trying to determine what dietary pattern is most likely to facilitate a long life without disease can be confusing. Nutrition science is difficult and conflicting at times. No topic generates more debate than the role of reducing dietary saturated fat for heart health. In the last few months, this situation has again grabbed headlines. Can you trust the new announcements that saturated fat was never a risk?

Research on the contribution of diets rich in saturated fats like cheese, butter, meats, eggs, and pastries to heart disease has been ongoing since the 1950's. Recently, a systematic review and meta-analysis of the relationship between saturated fat and heart disease was published by the Cochrane Database of Systematic Reviews (CDSR) on May 19, 2020. The CDSR is widely regarded as the leading and most respected of sources for evaluating topics in health care. The authors analyzed 15 controlled trials involving over 59,000 subjects and concluded that "The findings of this updated review suggest that reducing saturated fat intake for at least two years causes a potentially important reduction in combined cardiovascular events (21%). Replacing the energy from saturated fat with polyunsaturated fat or carbohydrate appear to be useful strategies." It would seem clear that reducing or eliminating meats, cheeses, egg yolks, lard, butter, ghee and baked goods would favor better odds of avoiding heart disease. You may have missed this important research paper as major media outlets did not report on this publication.

The CDSR lasted was buried by a publication that followed it by 4 weeks. A "State of the Art Review" by 12 authors on the topic of saturated fat and health was published in a major cardiology journal on June 16, 2020. They did not do original research, but rather analyzed previously published studies. The 12 authors concluded that "Whole-fat dairy, unprocessed meat, eggs and dark chocolate are SFA-rich foods with a complex matrix that are not associated with increased risk of CVD. The totality of available evidence does not support further limiting the intake of such foods." Unlike the esteemed CDSR paper, this review created 100's of headlines worldwide that implied enjoy your meats, cheeses, pastries and egg yolks again without concern.

How can we reconcile such conflicting conclusions? The media failed to report that the 2nd paper was written by authors with important funding conflicts of interest. Indeed, 9 of the 12 authors of the 2nd paper disclosed funding by dairy or beef foundations. At least 75% of the authors promoting saturated fat were funded by industry organizations that promote foods rich in saturated fat!

In a second challenge to the findings of the CDSR to reduced foods rich in saturated fats, 10 different authors published a "hypothesis" that those suffering from a relatively rare genetic disorder causing a high cholesterol would benefit more from a low-carbohydrate diet than a low-fat diet. The media, again, went wild reporting on this paper, but they left out that 5 of the 10 authors revealed financial ties that they benefit from relating to low-carb diets. The other 5 are well known low-carb advocates routinely advocating for dietary approaches in conflict with major medical societies and research findings.

When I am faced with conflicting data like these reports I rely on a structure for analyzing nutrition research proposed by Valter Longo, Ph.D, author of The Longevity Diet and creator of the plant-based Fasting Mimicking Diet. In his book, Longo favors the use of the "Five Pillars of Longevity" as a format to evaluate nutrition research.

These 5 pillars are: Biochemical research, Randomized trials, Epidemiology, Study of centenarians, and Analysis of complex systems (like the environmental impact of a diet).

Dr. Longo teaches a plant-based diet low in foods rich in saturated fat (e.g., no red meat or poultry) in his book as it encompasses all 5 pillars of science. Using the 5 Pillars of Longevity, there is ample data from biochemical studies, randomized trials, epidemiology, and centenarian data that indicate that diets lower in saturated fats improve health and reduce the risk of heart disease.

Simply put, 1-2 studies with severe funding conflicts cannot upend 70 years of high-quality research.

This is the good news, of course.

And in today's world, we think that journalism is dead and most of the political news is fake! This false narrative concept, it seems, is pervasive, even in the health industry where human lives are at stake. Mark Twain was right when he cautioned us: "...Beware, you may die of a misprint." If he were alive today, he would have also said, "Beware, you may die of misrepresentation."

We can say the same thing where medicines are pushed out by the pharma industry which gives funding to so-called experts to write articles in favor of their agendas and donate money to sway politicians for their advantage.

In addition to some of the health news fake media, there are other institutional entities one must fend against for survival and well-being (See Figure. 2.1. Medical Consumer Spider Web). For example, the food industry manipulation, political bureaucracy, one's cultural constraints, and so on. The individuals working in these organization entities are mostly well-meaning, hardworking people whom we respect and admire. The diagram has two aspects: the person as the medical consumer and the person as the victim. One is caught up in the web, and the other is a victim due to their own actions or lack thereof.

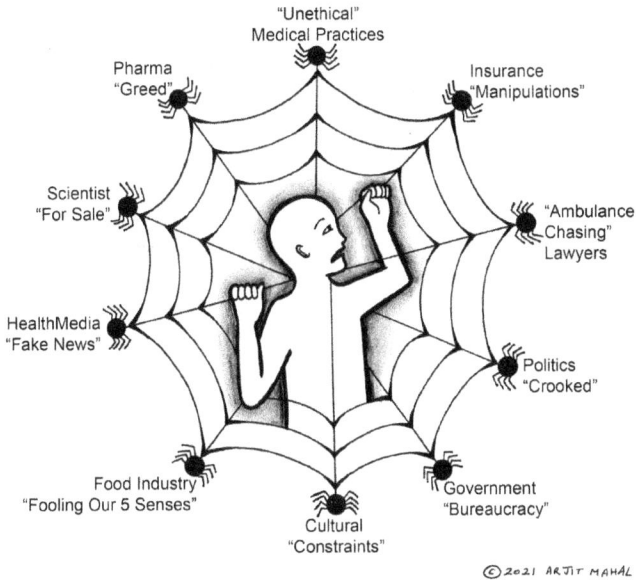

Figure 2.1 Medical Consumer Spider Web

The answer lies in self-responsibility.

Then who to trust?

Only yourself, your own "research," instincts and common sense.

Become a Self-Advocate for your own well-being.

I am the Primary Physician of my Body, My True Healer.

Arjit Mahal

As stated in the earlier chapter: know thyself, take charge. Take accountability for your understanding of your body's anatomy and systems which enable the body to work in such a wondrous way.

Do research on the internet, periodicals, read, read, read, and watch videos. Never in the history of the world have we had the capability to learn about our own health issues, their diagnosis, and potential solutions. Ensure that the research sources are reliable and authentic from reputable institutions and organizations such as Mayo Clinic, Cleveland Clinic, and governmental agencies such as FDA and CDC.

After reading contradictory information in many books and magazines and scanning websites, I decided to develop a thought framework. This framework is simply a collection of ideas, research, and philosophy of wise humans that helped shape my approach to decision-making for better health.

The definitions and images are my way of honoring those who have passed on their wisdom to us.

OCKHAM'S RAZOR[1], or Law of Parsimony, is the problem-solving principle which states that "entities should not be multiplied without necessity," or more simply, the simplest explanation is usually the right one. This idea is attributed to English Franciscan friar William of Ockham (c. 1287–1347), a philosopher and theologian who used a preference for simplicity to defend the idea of divine miracles. This approach advocates that when presented with competing hypotheses, one should select the solution with the fewest assumptions. This approach is not meant to be a way of choosing between theories that make different predictions.

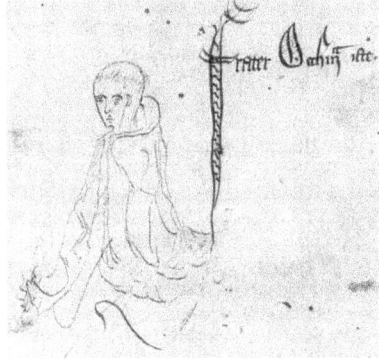

My Take: One Example - obesity may result in diabetes.

FOOD IS MEDICINE: Hippocrates of Kos (c. 460 – c. 370 BC), also known as Hippocrates II, was a Greek physician of the Age of Pericles (Classical Greece).

---

[1] Sketch labeled 'frater Occham iste', 1341, from a manuscript of Ockham's *Summa Logicae*, MS Gonville and Caius College, Cambridge, 464/571, fol. 69 Source: Wikimedia.org.

Hippocrates[2] is considered one of the most outstanding figures in the history of medicine. He is often referred to as the "Father of Medicine" to recognize his lasting contributions to the field as the founder of the Hippocratic School of Medicine. This intellectual school revolutionized Ancient Greek medicine, establishing it as a discipline distinct from other disciplines (theology and philosophy), thus establishing medicine as a profession.

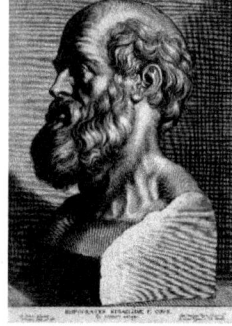

My Take: Mother-Earth-Diet may be the best medicine for me!

"TVAM BHUMIR APO, ANALO, ANILO, NABHA": You, The Supreme Lord alone are Earth, Water, Fire, Air, and Ether (Atmosphere). Ancient Sanskrit Wisdom.

Charaka[3] (Born c. 300 BC) was a noted Ayurveda practitioner who wrote the famous treatise on medicine *Charaka Samahita*. He wrote extensively on digestion, metabolism, and the immune system. According to Charaka, the body functions because it contains three *doshas* -

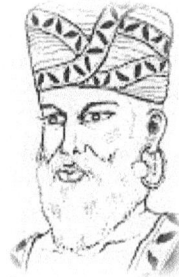

---

[2] Hippocrates - Wikipedia; Engraving by Peter Paul Rubens, 1638.

[3] www.thisismyindia.com. Engraving Charaka.

bile, phlegm, and wind. Consuming *dhatus* (blood, flesh, and marrow) produces doshas. The body becomes sick when there is an imbalance between the three doshas. Charaka cautions the physician who fails to enter a patient's body with the lamp of knowledge and understanding that they can never treat the disease. Charaka put more emphasis on prevention rather than cure.

My Take: Maintain harmony with nature; natural foods and earth, water, fire, air, and ether.

HOMEOSTASIS: A state of equilibrium, as in an organism or cell, maintained by self-regulating processes.

In biology, homeostasis is the state of steady internal, physical, and chemical conditions maintained by living systems. This is the condition of optimal functioning for the organism and includes many variables, such as body temperature and fluid balance, being kept within certain pre-set limits (homeostatic range). Other variables include the pH of extracellular fluid, the concentrations of sodium, potassium, and calcium ions, and the blood sugar level. These need to be regulated despite changes in the environment, diet, or level of activity. One or more regulators or homeostatic mechanisms control each of these variables, which together maintain life.

The concept of the regulation of the internal environment was described by French physiologist Claude Bernard in

1849, and the word *homeostasis* was coined by Walter Bradford Cannon in 1926. (He had also coined the term *fight or flight*.)

My Take: Example: Too much of something put in the body will resist e.g., overeating, sugar.

THE DOSE MAKES THE POISON: Anything can be harmful in excessive amounts, even if it is typically considered beneficial. (Paracelsus (1493-1541) A Swiss-German physician considered the founder of modern toxicology).

Paracelsus[4], a Renaissance physician, botanist, and alchemist, once noted, "Everything is poison, there is poison in everything." The danger of poison is in the dosage, he concluded. Some perilous substances are harmless in small doses, but anything can be toxic if you ingest or absorb enough. Paracelsus is the father of toxicology. His investigations brought a scientific analysis of toxins, and he forged the path of using chemicals and minerals in medicine.

---

[4] Source: ancient-origins.net, Portrait,1540 by Hirschvogel, during Paracelsus's lifetime.

My Take: Example: Insulin helps in managing diabetes but also causes obesity and increased insulin resistance.

AUTOPHAGY: The natural, regulated mechanism of the cell that removes unnecessary or dysfunctional components.

In 2016, the Nobel Assembly at Karolinska Institute awarded the Nobel Prize in Physiology or Medicine to Yoshinori Ohsumi[5] for his discoveries of mechanisms for autophagy. But what is autophagy? The word derives from the Greek auto (self) an *"phagein"* (to eat). So, the word literally means to eat oneself. Essentially, this is the body's mechanism of getting rid of all the broken down, old cell machinery (organelles, proteins, and cell membranes) when there is no longer enough energy to sustain it. It is a regulated, orderly process to degrade and recycle cellular components.

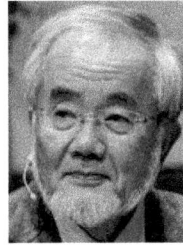

My Take: Weight loss causes body cells to "dump" fat and makes them healthier/efficient.

---

[5] Reference: Dr-Jason-Fung–The Epoch theepoch.org. Yoshinori Ohsumi-Wikipedia en.wikipedia.org.

"MAN JEETA JAG-JEET": When you win over your mind, you win the world! (Guru Nanak Ji, 1469-1539, Gurmukhi: ਗੁਰੂ ਨਾਨਕ).

The founder of the Sikh Philosophical thought, Guru Nanak's message is **Naam, Daan, Insaan**: *Naam* (Mindful Awareness of Divine Presence)[6], *Daan* (Live Out the Culture of Altruism when Seeking Divine Benevolence), *Isnaan* (Through love for all nature, implement ethics of good deeds that cleanse both body and mind). His divine message was: The Creator is ONE, Accept What is!

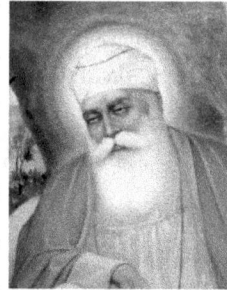

My Take: Mind Over Matter – Needed for self-transformation of health and well-being.

---

[6] Image Source: SikhNet, Sobha Singh Painting.

CHAPTER 3

Digestive System

One man's food is another man's poison.

Lucretius

D r. Jason Fung, in his book, *The Obesity Code, Unlocking the Secrets of Weight Loss.* Greystone Books 2016., describes food digestion thus:

"Whole foods can be divided into three different macronutrient groups: fat, protein, and carbohydrates. The "macro" in "macronutrients" refers to the fact that the bulk of the food we eat comprises these three groups. Micronutrients, which make up a tiny proportion of the food, include vitamins A, B, C, D, E, and K and minerals such as iron and calcium. Starchy foods and sugars are all carbohydrates. A calorie is simply a unit of energy. Burn different foods in a laboratory, and the amount of heat released is measured to determine a caloric value for that food. (Per Dr. J. Aujla, there are close to 3,500 calories in a pound. Imagine how long it would take to burn those on a treadmill but how fast it would be ingesting those through cake!)

How do we process food? All the foods we eat contain calories. Food first enters the stomach, where it mixes with acid. Then the processing food is slowly released into the small intestine. Nutrients are extracted throughout the journey through the small and large intestines. Lastly, what remains is excreted as stool."

This chapter describes these two processes as an outline because these body parts and concepts appear in the rest of the book: *The Digestive System and The Blood Glucose Homeostasis.*

The Digestive System turns the food you eat into nutrients, which the body uses for energy, growth, and cell repair. Additionally, this system is the source of numerous disorders yet can also prevent diseases and thus enable healing through its symbiotic relationship with other systems such as the body's immune system.

In their book, *The Whole-Body Micro Biome, How to Harness Microbes Inside and Out—for Lifelong Health,* B. Brett Finlay, Ph.D. and Jessica M. Finlay, Ph.D., write: "The mouth reflects overall health at any stage of life and represents the critical first contact between our alimentary (the gastrointestinal tract along which food passes from mouth to anus), the immune system, and the outside world. If we envision the gastrointestinal tract as a river, the mouth is the source: the headwaters from which everything flows downstream. In fact, the majority of all systemic diseases (those involving many organs or the whole body) produce oral signs and symptoms…your mouth is a window into the condition of your entire body and can serve as a critical vantage point to detect and defend against problems."

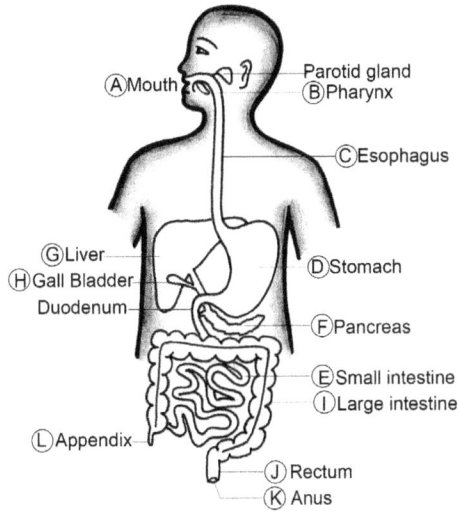

© 2021 ARJIT MAHAL

Figure 3.1 Human Digestive System

- **Mouth.** The mouth is the beginning of the digestive tract. Chewing breaks the food while saliva mixes it to begin the process of absorption.

- **Throat.** Also called the pharynx, the throat is the next destination for food you've eaten. From here, food travels to the esophagus or swallowing tube.

- **Esophagus.** A muscular tube extending from the pharynx to the stomach. By means of a series of contractions, called peristalsis, the esophagus delivers food to the stomach.

- **Stomach.** The stomach secretes acid and powerful enzymes that continue the process of breaking down the food. When it leaves the stomach, food is the consistency of a liquid or paste. As the food enters the small intestine, the liver, pancreas, and gallbladder work in conjunction to free the nutrients. Both the gallbladder and pancreas have drains to the first part of your intestine (duodenum). Their enzymes escalate the breakdown process the stomach started.

- **Small Intestine.** Made up of three segments, the duodenum, jejunum, and ileum, the small intestine is a long tube loosely coiled in the abdomen (spread out, it would be more than 20 feet long). The duodenum is largely responsible for continuing the process of breaking down food, with the jejunum and ileum being mainly responsible for the absorption of nutrients into the bloodstream.

- **Large Intestine.** This is a five- to six-foot-long muscular tube wider than the small intestine and continues the journey of your food. Water is removed from the food, and the once-liquid consistency will now form to become stool.

Blood Glucose Homeostasis

Blood Glucose Homeostasis has interrelated biological processes which manage the harmony between blood glucose, insulin, and glucagon. The main organs immediately involved in this process are the pancreas, liver, and insulin hormone. Of course, these are within the purview of the digestive system and in the context of numerous other body organs and processes. The solid organs have multiple functions. The enzymes secreted by the gallbladder and pancreas to the intestine/duodenum are different from the insulin-producing function of the pancreas.

Figure 3.2, Blood Glucose Homeostasis, is a conceptual view as envisioned by me to ease my learning. (Ideas sourced from public domain.) The objective of this diagram is to give a high-level understanding of what happens when the body continuously tries to maintain its glucose levels and the resulting energy disbursement.

When we eat, the Beta Cells of the pancreas stimulate the release of insulin into the bloodstream. Glucose released through the actions of the acidic breakdown creates energy. Insulin serves as a shuttle for the glucose to get to where it's needed. The liver takes the extra glucose and stores it as glycogen. After the blood glucose level declines to a setpoint, the stimulus of insulin declines.

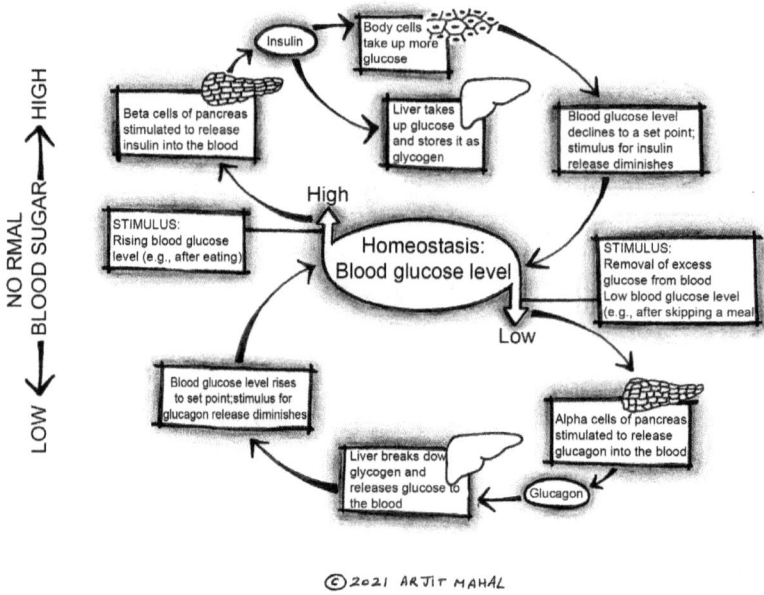

Figure 3.2 Blood Glucose Homeostasis

When we do not eat or skip a meal, as an example, other cells in the pancreas mobilize the glycogen, and the liver converts it back to glucose—to use as energy. The blood glucose levels rise to get to a setpoint, and the stimulus of the glycogen release diminishes. Homeostasis facilitates the see-saw of balance. This all is, of course, a normal process scenario underway all the time. The understanding of the processes equips us with better tools to manage our overall health—particularly diabetes.

CHAPTER 4

Diabetes

He is the best physician who is the most ingenious inspirer of hope.

Samuel Taylor Coleridge (1772-1834)

This chapter on diabetes is not a tutorial or a complete medical education on this topic. It is only for what I have learned for myself to embark upon the initiative of reversing[7] diabetes. Diabetes is a progressive disease that can damage just about all parts of the body if not effectively managed and controlled.

My quest to "reverse" this disease and my heart disease, discussed in the next chapter, is not necessarily to increase my life span. Instead, I hope to have a reasonable quality

---

[7] The meaning of the term reverse, reversing, reversal, from the Online Dictionary, Copyright 2020, Merriam-Webster, Incorporated: movement in reverse, to undo or negate the effect of, opposite or contrary to a previous or normal condition, to turn or move in the opposite direction, an act or the process of reversing.

of life and living for whatever time I have left on this earth. I am a positive-minded individual and enjoy the gift of life given to me by nature.

In this chapter, I describe the genesis of my diabetes condition, the progressive state of increased medications, and my experience with what I could or could not learn from the medical practitioners. The hope came to me by some books—which put me on a track to success.

For reference, here are abbreviated descriptions provided by Dr. J. Aujla for some of the medications I used to take: Metformin stops the liver from storing and releasing glycogen/glucose. Glimepiride stimulates your pancreas to make more insulin. Insulin helps the pancreas meet the body's insulin demand. There are other medications too, but they are too complex for this discussion, yet all end up trying to decrease glucose into your bloodstream.

My Diabetes Timeline Diary

2005 (16 years ago). Diagnosed with Diabetes type 2. Started one oral medication (Metformin). Dose kept on increasing over the years to ensure glucose numbers were in the prescribed range. Attended diabetes nutrition programs for learning to eat what, when, and how. Outcome: A new challenge to manage nature's hand of cards dealt to me in the form of diabetes.

2013-2016 - 3 Years. Additional oral medications were added, which off and on included: Glimpride, Tanzeum, Onglyza, etc. Outcome: Continued to struggle with keeping A1c within range (less than 6%).

2018 January. Started Insulin Regimen. Humalog (short-acting) three times a day: before breakfast 11 IUs (International Units), before lunch, 15 IUs and before dinner 25 IUs; and Tresiba (long-acting 20-24 IUs) before bed. Total Insulin IUs taken approximately 70 to 80 in a day (Not considered "very high" dose measured against my weight in kilograms). My weight increased from 174 to 190 Lbs (16 Lbs) by mid-2019. Just about one pound would increase every month despite my exercise and better diet regimen. Outcome: Not happy with the overweight. A1c was better managed, however.

2019 July. My endocrinologist introduced and prescribed a CGM, the Continuous Glucose Monitoring tool. This has a sensor that is like a patch with a needle, placed on the upper arm for 14 days before replacing. The blood glucose can be checked at any time with a monitor. This monitor has a mass of relevant data for effectively managing your diabetes numbers (more on this in Chapter 9: Tools). Outcome: Stopped pricking figures to test my blood glucose (what a relief!). The CGM tool became a game changer in my glucose management.

2019 September. Read Dr. Neal Barnard's book: *Program for Reversing Diabetes, The Scientifically Proven System for Reversing Diabetes Without Drugs*, Rodale Books 2017. Being mostly vegetarian in my diet, this book's proposed plant-based, no animal products diet appealed to me. I started to follow the program on my own. I called Dr. Barnard's clinic to get guidance, but due to the pandemic constraint I was not successful in getting access to their advisors at that time, and they did not have a license to practice in New Jersey. Outcome: My weight started to drop, and my need for insulin began to come down. I was pleased with the progress.

2020 Jan-June - 6 months. I learned about the Autophagy process, which, through fasting, enables the body to clear glucose clogged body cells and makes the insulin more effective, resulting in a reduction in insulin resistance (see Chapter 8: Fasting).

I read Dr. Jason Fung's book: *The Diabetes Code, Prevent and Reverse Type 2 Diabetes Naturally*, Greystone Books 2016. This book's approach added more enthusiasm for me on the plant-based food diet (but some good fats are allowed). Outcome: Dr. Fung's fasting regimen appealed to me. So, I started fasting—on my own. I had called Dr. Fung's clinic in Toronto for consultation. I was told that Dr. Fung does not see patients. So, I was on my own. My weight had dropped from 190 to about 180 pounds.

2020 July-September - 3 Months. In May, I had an angina condition that resulted in the discovery of a blockage in one area, called stenosis, the pathological narrowing of a passage. Stents were placed for a third time in the same place. Sponsored by his practice, The Hunterdon Cardiovascular Associates, my cardiologist Dr. Harnish Chawla prescribed that I attend a nine-week reversing heart disease program at the Hunterdon Cardiac Rehab Department of the Hunterdon Medical Center in Flemington, NJ. Based on Dr. Dean Ornish's research, this program is called the *Ornish Lifestyle Medicine* Reversing Heart Disease Program. The program has four related and symbiotic concepts: Nutrition, Fitness, Stress Management, and Support. The Cardiac Rehab's multidisciplinary competent staff coached and trained me along with other enrollees in all four aspects—in a way to make it a lifelong habit (more on this in Chapter 5: The Heart).

Outcome: The Ornish Program was another game-changer in the management of my diabetes and heart health, as well as weight management. My weight had dropped to about 170 pounds. My waist shrunk by four inches. I felt much healthier overall. My need for insulin had dropped from four times a day to once a day at a low dose.

2020 October – December. I continued a plant-based diet, the Ornish Lifestyle Medicine practice, and fasting. Outcome: Stopped Insulin (most of it), except one small dose of insulin to manage post-meal spike. My weight started to drop and came down to 164 pounds by October 10. When I exercised about 30 to 40 minutes a day, no insulin was needed. However, I had to curtail my exercise for unrelated reasons, which resulted in an ad hoc intake of insulin. So, during this period, I could not say that I had stopped 100% of medication, but it had dropped down to about 15% to 20% of the peak of two years.

Timeline Thoughts

For the past 15 years, no medical practitioner nor any diabetic nutritionist ever once mentioned to me that diabetes can be reversed, reduced, or put in remission—whatever term may be preferred. When I had mentioned to my doctor that I have reversed diabetes, the doctor was prompt to respond that diabetes cannot be reversed and stated that what I was doing was Diet Managed Diabetes!

For 15 years, I was under the care of three different endocrinology practices. While they were qualified and I respected their training in this science and their advice about good diet and exercise, no one said that there is a possibility of "reversing" diabetes. In fact, I made a copy of Dr. Neil Barnard's book's title page to show to one of my doctors. The doctor did not even take the copy from my hand and simply brushed off by saying, "authors want to sell books!" Yet another one showed interest and took the copy from me. There are, of course, some physicians, as in any profession, who invest in their self-development.

My Understanding of Diabetes

My narrative contains direct quotes from experts such as Dr. Neil Barnard. He wrote a book on reversing diabetes, which became my master reference book, particularly for initiating my journey on a plant-based diet to "reverse" diabetes.[8] Based on important research findings, Dr. Neil Barnard proposed a new approach, a revolutionary method for preventing, controlling, and reversing diabetes. This approach opened my eyes to the possibility of hope.

The prevailing notion was 'once you have diabetes, you'll always have diabetes,' and the condition just seemed to lead to more and more complications. We have changed that scenario.

Dr. Neil Barnard

His method is on changing the diet and not the drugs. However, the drugs may still be needed to some extent, but they also can be eliminated entirely. He is clear that

---

[8] Barnard, Neal D. Dr. *Program for Reversing Diabetes, the Scientifically Proven System for Reversing Diabetes Without Drugs*. RodaleBooks 2017. Pages: xi – xiii.

one does not have to cut calories or even limit carbohydrates and food portions in his eating approach.

In a critical analysis that kept exercise and medication use constant, we found that the new diet-controlled blood sugar three times more effectively than the previous 'best' diet. It also accelerates weight loss and controls cholesterol better than the old gold standard.

Dr. Neil Barnard

For the goal of managing my blood sugar (diabetes), losing weight, and cholesterol control (heart-related healing), this proposed idea of "reversing diabetes" was a "light at the end of the long tunnel" opportunity. My transformation had begun. Most people with diabetes find themselves on the road to increasing weight, doses of medications, and resulting complications.

If weight is an issue, it can come down gradually, but decisively. Blood glucose values that have gone up can also come down. Doses of medications that have risen again and again can come down, too. Symptoms such as neuropathy-- nerve pain in the feet and legs--can improve and even disappear. Heart disease can be reversed.

Dr. Neil Barnard

No doctor ordered a C-Peptide test until about two years ago when my endocrinologist ordered this test. The test showed that my pancreas produces insulin, but the insulin autoantibodies are attacking my insulin-producing cells. It was then when my doctor changed the diagnosis classification to type 1.5, LADA. I now understand that doctors sometimes misdiagnose type 1.5 as type 2 diabetes.

Your body needs the hormone insulin to move sugar through your bloodstream to your cells for energy. A healthy pancreas makes equal amounts of insulin and the protein C-peptide. By measuring your C-peptide, your healthcare provider can also learn about your insulin level. Measuring C-peptide can show whether you have type 1 or type 2 diabetes. In type 1 diabetes, your body does not make any insulin. In type 2 diabetes, either your body does not make enough insulin, or your cells cannot use it normally. If you have diabetes the C-peptide test can show how well your treatment is working.

University of Rochester Medical Center
Health Encyclopedia, www.urmc.rochester.edu

In my case, type 1.5, also called LADA (Latent Autoimmune Diabetes in Adults), means that my pancreas is producing insulin, but my own insulin antibodies are attacking it in a "friendly fire" scenario. I also have insulin resistance. Therefore, I have a double whammy: insulin deficiency because of type 1.5 and insulin resistance because of type 2 diabetes. In a later chapter, I note that after successfully reducing my weight, my C-Peptide test showed that my own pancreas had started to make more insulin. What I can do about the autoantibodies is my next challenge. If I can do something about it, I could possibly reverse diabetes altogether.

For more information on diabetes, including an overview of the different types, please refer to The Centers of Disease Control and Prevention's (CDC) website: https://www.cdc.gov/diabetes/basics/diabetes.html.

The fundamental problem is that sugar is not able to pass from your bloodstream into the cells of your body. The sugar we are speaking of is glucose…if glucose is unable to enter your cells, they are deprived of their basic fuel, so you lose your energy…When you change your diet and make other help helpful improvements, a rising glucose level can fall. Sometimes the change can be so dramatic that no doctors looking at you afterward ever guess that you had once been diagnosed with diabetes.

Dr. Neil Barnard

What is Insulin Resistance? Unlike type 1 diabetes, where due to autoimmune reaction, the body does not make enough insulin and diabetics need to take it to survive, type 2 diabetes is insulin-resistant. Billions of the body's cells cannot absorb the glucose in the bloodstream and convert it into energy for the body's organs. Another way to state this is that the cells are not insulin sensitive.

The Centers of Disease Control and Prevention (CDC) explains insulin resistance here: https://bit.ly/3h6HSDp. Since the terms Insulin, Glucagon, and Glycogen appear in many places in this and subsequent chapters, here is a short description with a visual to understand their relationship with the pancreas. The conceptual diagram in Figure 4.1 Pancreas and Liver shows a physical view of the stomach, pancreas, liver, and intestines.

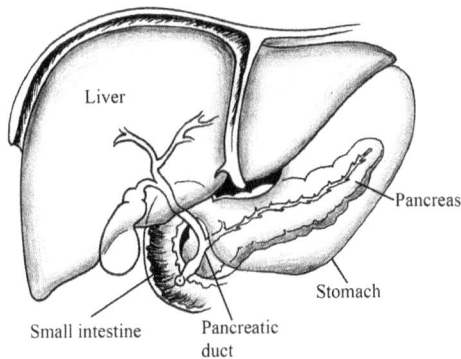

Figure 4.1 Pancreas and Liver[9]

Insulin is a hormone produced by the beta cells of the pancreas. When food is eaten, these cells secrete insulin into the bloodstream to be taken to the body's cells for energy conversion. Glucagon is also a hormone which plays a vital role in regulating blood glucose concentration

---

[9] Inspired by the graphic from https://wb.md/3x8FZf7. Human Anatomy By Matthew Hoffman, MD. Image Source© 2014 WebMD, LLC.

when it is lower than default level, but the glycogen is a form of storage compound in human and other animals. Glucagon is synthesized by the alpha cells of the pancreas, while glycogen is synthesized and stored in the liver. Glucagon helps to convert glycogen into glucose, when necessary.

Insulin Resistance Conceptual Process

Figure 4.2 contains the author's view of the Insulin Resistance Conceptual Process in three scenarios: a normal person and type 2 and type 1.5 diabetics.

In a non-diabetic person, as the food is being digested, the pancreas produces insulin, which along with the blood stream, opens the cell receptors of billions of cells. There, metabolization of glucose and fat particles occurs, and energy is generated and sent to the muscles and other parts of the body. In a type 2 diabetic, the cells' receptors inhibit glucose and its facilitator insulin from entering the cells. The insulin and glucose build up—thereby causing the glucose to reverse into the bloodstream. This, in simple terms, is insulin resistance. And simply put, excessive insulin resistance promotes weight gain. In type 1.5 (LADA) diabetics, there is the additional constraint where there is a low level of insulin produced by the pancreas due to the autoimmune destruction of the insulin-producing cells.

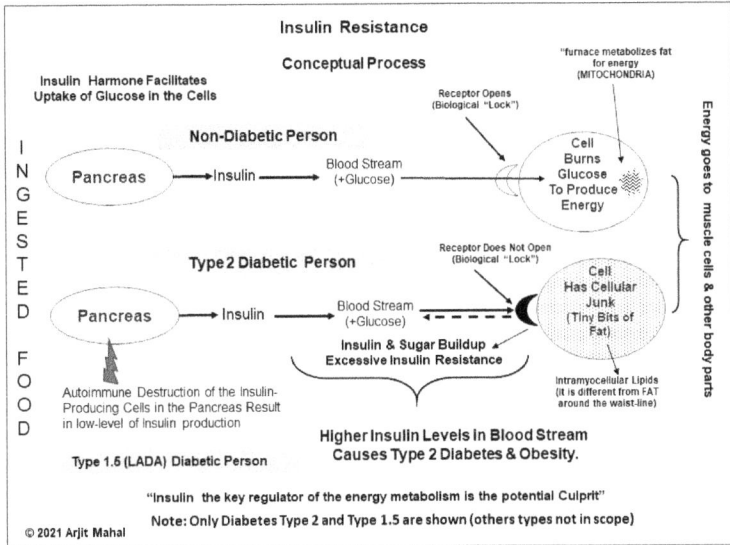

Figure 4.2 Insulin Resistance Conceptual Process

Healthy Diet and Lifestyle

After reading Dr. Neil Barnard's book, I was convinced that I should follow his suggestion of plant-based foods. Dr. Dean Ornish's Lifestyle Medicine program later confirmed this. I strongly advise those interested in managing their diabetes to "invest" in buying Dr. Barnard's book for a detailed understanding of the research and science behind such a simple yet effective approach for managing type 2 diabetes and for general health and wellbeing.

For people on a plant-based diet, among many other things written in his book, Dr. Barnard recommends Vitamin B12 and Vitamin D. From my experience, I have created a visual to describe what happened with my glucose management after being on a plant-based diet, the Ornish Lifestyle Medicine program, and fasting, which I will cover in subsequent chapters on heart and fasting.

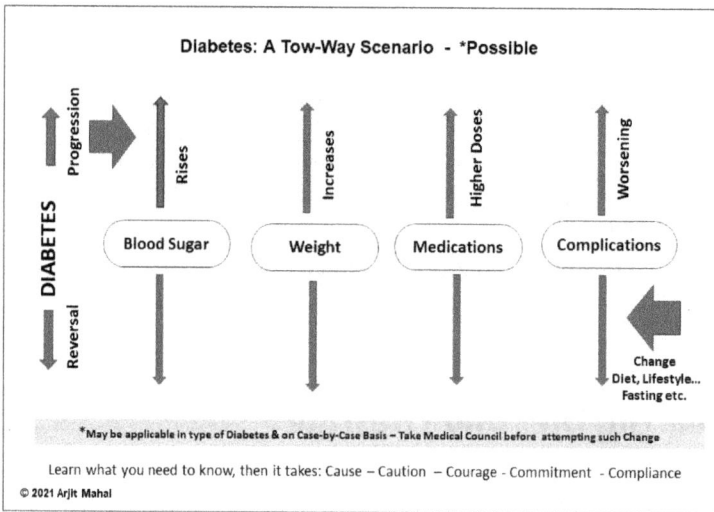

Figure 4.3 Diabetes A Two-Way Scenario – Possible

Fifteen years ago, when I was diagnosed with type 2 diabetes, I was put on the basic medication Metformin. Later, over time when the glucose numbers were not getting in the desired range, more medications were added, one after the other, until my doctor decided that I should be on insulin.

Reference the upper half of Figure 4.3. As the blood glucose (sugar) rises or is not managed well, the weight increases, and higher doses of medications are taken, thus setting the stage for worsening health complications. While I did not have related health complications such as with my eyes, I had a serious concern as a heart patient. After changing my diet and lifestyle, I experienced the "two-way" scenario as seen in the bottom half of Figure 4.3. My dentist noted that my gums were more "pink" and healthier and my heart blood profile became better than it was ever before to the best of my memory. The medication doses had to be lowered or eliminated, such as the blood pressure medication. My weight had dropped dramatically, and I was able to manage my glucose numbers better.

Thus, for me, the progression of diabetes was reversed. It works! Everybody's body and medical conditions vary. While the general guidelines for glucose numbers are a good standard marker, each person should study their own situation—in addition to the conventional wisdom. For example, prior to going on fasting, my A1c was 6.7%, but after reversing the diabetes, my A1c was 7.1%. The prior number was when I was taking insulin four times a day, and the later number is the one when I had stopped taking insulin. (**Note also that the numbers may differ by**

ethnicity. Read the *diaTribe* December 24, 2020, article diatribe.org).

My Reference Guide for Glucose Measures

God built the universe on Numbers; Numbers rule the universe.

Pythagoras, Greek philosopher and mathematician

Disclaimer: The measures and the associated numbers outlined here are for my need and reference only. The list does not imply priority. Anyone interested in knowing about their own unique needs must consult their medical professionals. To ensure that I monitor my blood glucose and thus monitor my health diligently, I started to track the relevant measures outlined below. The reports of some of these critical numbers are discussed in Chapter 9: Tools.

I use the following charts for reference to monitor my glucose status: Reference: American Diabetes Association. https://diabetes.org. If your A1C level is between 5.7 and 6.5%, your levels are in the prediabetes range. If you have an A1C level of 6.5% or higher, your levels are in the diabetes range.

Fasting	
Normal for person without diabetes	70–99 mg/dl (3.9–5.5 mmol/L)
Official ADA recommendation for someone with diabetes	80–130 mg/dl (4.4–7.2 mmol/L)
1 to 2 hours after meals	
Normal for person without diabetes	Less than 140 mg/dl (7.8 mmol/L)
Official ADA recommendation for someone with diabetes	Less than 180 mg/dl (10.0 mmol/L)
HbA1c	
Normal for person without diabetes	Less than 5.7%
Official ADA recommendation for someone with diabetes	Less than 7.0%

Table 4.1 Blood Glucose Chart. Source: diabetesselfmanagement.com

A1C	eAG	
%	mg/dl milligrams per deciliter	Mmol/l Millimoles per liter
6	126	7.0
6.5	140	7.8
7.0	154	8.6
7.5	169	9.4
8	183	10.1
8.5	197	10.9
9	212	11.8
9.5	226	12.6
10	240	13.4

Table 4.2 Comparison of A1C and eAG readings. Source: American Diabetes Association.

My Glucose Monitoring List

1. Daily Glucose Numbers at various times in the day: before meals and after meals, also known as post-prandial (after meal) blood glucose spike.

2. *A1c:* hemoglobin A1c or HbA1c test: a simple blood test that measures your average blood sugar levels over the past three months. A1c test results are reported as a percentage; the higher the percentage, the higher your blood sugar levels over the past two to three months.

3. *eAG* (Estimated Average Glucose): helps people with diabetes better understand how their A1c results compare to their daily glucose readings and shows how well you are controlling your diabetes.

4. *TIR* ("Time in Range"): is the percentage of time that a person spends with their blood glucose levels in a target range. General guidelines suggest starting with a range of 70 to 180 mg/dl and then aim for a tighter range—suggested by one's physician.

5. Awareness of glucose numbers' fluctuation at nighttime and upon waking up in the morning: Somogyi Effect and Dawn Phenomenon.

For people who have diabetes, the Somogyi effect and the dawn phenomenon both cause higher blood sugar levels in the morning. The body uses glucose as its main source of energy. While you sleep, your body doesn't need as much energy. But when you're about to wake up, it gets ready to burn more fuel. It tells your liver to start releasing more glucose into your blood. That should trigger your body to release more insulin to handle more blood sugar. If you have diabetes, your body doesn't make enough insulin to do that. That leaves too much sugar in your blood, a problem called hyperglycemia.

If you have diabetes, your body doesn't release more insulin to match the early-morning rise in blood sugar. It's called the dawn phenomenon, since it usually happens between 3 a.m. and 8 a.m. The Somogyi effect also causes high levels of blood sugar in the early morning. But it usually happens when you take too much or too little insulin before bed, or when you skip your nighttime snack. When that happens, your blood sugar can drop sharply overnight. Your body responds by releasing hormones that work against insulin. That means you'll have too much blood sugar in the morning. It's also called rebound hyperglycemia.

WebMD: www.webmd.com

Summary

After reading Dr. Barnard's book, I was convinced that I must start a total plant-based diet. I was still unsure about eating preferences, including nuts, eggs, and fruit. Nuts have healthy fat, but another study shows to keep those to a minimum. While Dr. Barnard writes that one should eliminate the entire egg, both the white and the yolk, some other authors show that white egg is okay; and yet other experts have said that the whole egg is good for diabetics. In Chapter 7: Nutrition, I go more into this dilemma. Similarly, nuts such as walnuts have natural fat and are considered good for the heart; however, some doctors advise limiting the quantity.

With a total plant-based diet, I started to lose weight and my need for insulin decreased dramatically. My weight started to drop. I started to feel better overall.

My transformation of health had begun!

My next step was to deal with my heart health.

The Heart

Scope: This chapter on the heart is not a tutorial or a complete medical education on this topic. My primary condition has been Coronary Artery Disease (CAD). Whereas CHD is a catch-all phrase for various conditions that affect the heart's structure and function, coronary heart disease is a type of heart disease that develops when the arteries of the heart cannot deliver enough oxygen-rich blood to the heart. My focus on reversing heart disease is based on my condition only: Coronary Artery Disease. Other specific heart-related issues are out of scope.

Conceptual/Partial Diagram of My Heart

Figure 5.1, My Heart Diagram, is a high-level view of my arteries which had had procedures performed on them since 1996. LIMA, the Left Internal Mammary Artery, is the bypass that has been open for the last 24 years. (Thanks to my then surgeon, late Dr. Gregory Scott, and his staff.) The other two areas are where stents had been placed, in some cases more than once.

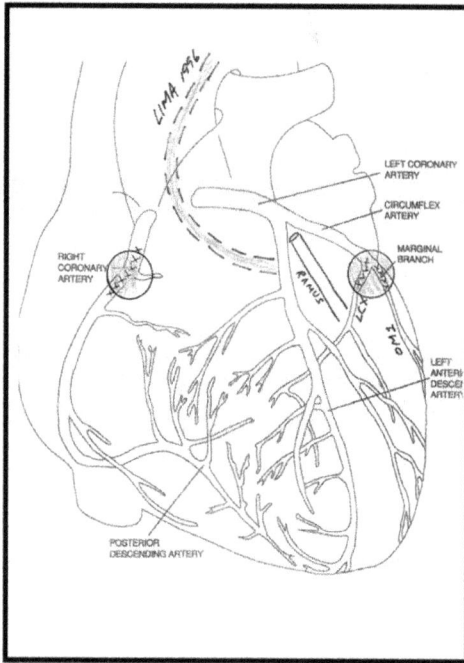

Figure 5.1 My Heart Diagram

I had to undergo a heart bypass surgery called CABG (Coronary Artery Bypass Grafting) in 1996 when I was only 48 years old. According to The Mayo Clinic:[10]

---

[10] © 1998-2020 Mayo Foundation for Medical Education and Research.

Coronary bypass surgery redirects blood around a section of a blocked or partially blocked artery in your heart. The procedure involves taking a healthy blood vessel from your leg, arm, or chest and connecting it below and above the blocked arteries in your heart. With a new pathway, blood flow to the heart muscle improves. Coronary bypass surgery doesn't cure the heart disease that caused the blockages, such as atherosclerosis or coronary artery disease. However, it can ease symptoms, such as chest pain and shortness of breath. For some people, this procedure can improve heart function and reduce the risk of dying of heart disease.

The Mayo Clinic

It is a wake-up call! One thinks about "why me?" and "Why at a relatively younger age did I have this event?" Many such thoughts crossed my mind. I felt a sort of minor depression on occasion—thinking about my whole life and personal and professional journey that remained ahead—with this condition accompanying me. I then started to do introspection, looking within as to what does this all means and how do I move on with the remainder of my journey of life.

As we know, heart conditions can be caused by many factors, stress being one of them. In the preceding five years, I had gone through a lot of issues due to family politics, which I believe were contributing factors in my case. I was convinced that stress had caused this issue. By deceit, to grab our parent's assets and exclude me from their will, two of my younger siblings had relentlessly destroyed my good relations with them. While I did not care about any assets, I valued their relationship more; I did not handle the whole process and the stress well. After expunging these siblings' relationships from my life— forever—I came up with my own plan to deal with stress. So, as an analyst, I started to identify some principles that can help me understand "what is" and what do I do so that a new chapter could begin with a positive attitude.

I had listed all the things personal and professional that I considered changing to move forward, including getting rid of toxic people from my life for good, lessening stressful things, and focusing on what matters most. I concluded that the quantity of remaining life is of no consequence; what matters most is the quality of the remainder of my life—whatever it may be. I came up with the following mantra to apply both in my personal and professional life.

Professional

I came up with the acronym **STOP**. This, I created as *a* mantra to be meditated upon daily in the morning and even repeating during the day as needed. I meditated on the STOP mantra and repeated those statements to myself every morning. During the day, if I faltered on one of these items, I would say "oh well" and meditate again upon these words. Eventually, these concepts become a habit.

S No short fuse today (meaning I would not get angry and "lose it," as I used to get sometimes).

T No time deadlines (I would schedule too many work-related activities back-to-back). This was a reminder not to do that.

O No oversensitivity (I had been an overly sensitive person; little things would bother me). This was a reminder to let go of issues that don't matter.

P No perfectionism (I used to be a perfectionist in everything, thus bringing stress upon myself). Everything does not have to be perfect; except heart surgery, brain surgery, or flying a jumbo jet, and such! Even nature is not perfect!

Table 5.1 Stress Management Mantra - Professional

In addition, I had sought other therapies which could help my heart. In a strange way, the CABG event became a blessing in disguise because my attitude and approach changed because of these mantras. This mantra helped me for many years to follow.

Personal

Harmony with Nature	Acceptance of "What Is" (not to dwell on what could have been and what could be).
Invest in Mutuality	Blood is thicker than water is a nonsense concept—most of the time. I believe that true relationships exist between individuals and groups where there is a mutuality of respect. And that is where I would invest my energy.
Let Go!	Everything is not to be taken too seriously. Be selective with what to focus on and what to let go of.

Table 5.2 Stress Management Mantra - Personal

My Heart Health Timeline Diary

Note: I have left some of the technical, medical terms for the benefit of medical practitioner readers.

1996: CABG Heart Bypass Surgery in December 1996; Procedure: LIMA to LAD Graft (LIMA: Left Internal Mammary Artery; LAD, Left Anterior Descending artery); A Saphenous Vein Graft (from the leg) to OM2 of the Circumflex (this graft was found blocked again in 2016 and 2019).

2008 to 2016: Angiography and Angioplasties performed in some arteries; in March 2008, May 2008, and 2016. Note:

Collateral Arteries Blood Supply was observed by the cardiologist.

2019 March: Diagnosis: Atherosclerotic heart disease Atherosclerosis refers to the buildup of fats, cholesterol, and other substances in and on your artery walls (plaque), which can restrict blood flow of native coronary artery without angina pectoris (angina pectoris is the medical term for chest pain or discomfort due to coronary heart disease). Intervention of the arteries: Circumflex: the proximal circumflex lesion was treated: The proximal LCX and the OM1 were simultaneously stented, creating a new crux. (LCX left circumflex artery or circumflex artery, or circumflex branch of the left coronary artery).

2020 May: Angina episode. Interventional catheterization was done in the same general area where the procedure was done twice earlier. Diagnosis: Stenosis: Constriction or narrowing of a passage. RAMUS: The left main coronary artery bifurcates into two or three vessels (LAD, LCX, Ramus). Following this third-time intervention, I wondered what if a blockage happens in the same area again—what would be my options. I had consulted two of the top heart surgeons in the country. They both assured me that should the blockage happen again; I could be a candidate for bypass-redo surgery (In their language, I have the "targets" available). This, for sure, was a comforting feeling to know that it may not be the end of the road yet! Since then, I have learned of yet another option: Brachytherapy, a form of radiotherapy radiation treatment. I hope I don't have to go to these options.

2020 July-Sept: Participated in *Ornish Lifestyle Medicine*: nine-week reversing heart disease program, based on Dr. Dean Ornish's "Undo-it" Approach, which includes awareness, training, and coaching in nutrition, fitness, stress management, and group support.

2020 Oct Onwards: Continued with a plant-based diet, Ornish Lifestyle Medicine Practice and Fasting, with a promising and positive outcome for my overall health.

In May 2020, after my latest procedure, my cardiologist, Dr. Harnish Chawla, a member of the Hunterdon Cardiovascular Associates Group in Flemington, New Jersey, had written a prescription and recommended that I participate in Ornish Lifestyle Medicine Program for reversing heart disease.

Added on to my plant-based diet and some fasting effort underway—on my own. **This prescription was a game-changer for my future well-being.**

Hunterdon Healthcare has a Cardiopulmonary Rehabilitation Department, which offers this nine-week program under the supervision of trained and competent staff that includes all four aspects of Ornish Lifestyle Medicine: Nutrition, Stress Management, Fitness, Love, and Support. I had attended a couple of other cardiac rehab programs over the years; this is different and transformational. This program is directed under the supervision of the Hunterdon Cardiovascular Associates and delivered by the Hunterdon Cardiac and Pulmonary Department of Hunterdon Healthcare, Flemington, New Jersey (https://www.hunterdonhealthcare.org/).

The following information appears on the Dean Ornish Lifestyle Medicine Website.[11]

> Ornish Lifestyle Medicine is more than a diet; it is a lifestyle. This lifestyle prescribes a plant-based diet that is naturally low in fat and includes exercise, stress management, and group support to maximize the many benefits of healthy living. Even a little movement in this direction can lower your blood sugar and help to prevent diabetes.

The first program has been scientifically proven to "undo" (reverse) heart disease by optimizing four important areas of your life. Participants experience the program within a small, consistent group, and all have the common goal of reversing their heart disease and improving their well-being. Each session lasts four hours, for a total of 72 hours. See Figure 5.2.

---

[11] https://www.ornish.com/. Copyright © 2020 Ornish Lifestyle Medicine. All rights reserved. Dean Ornish, MD Digital Magazine; Contact Us +1 (877) 888-3091.

What you eat ---   *How you manage stress*

How much you move   *How much love & support you have*

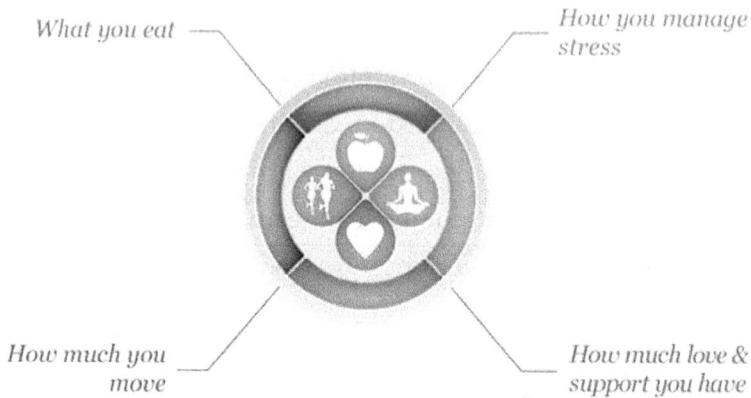

Figure 5.2 Ornish Lifestyle Medicine Model

The Difference: This program has been proven to undo heart disease by dealing with the root causes and not just its effects. The combined effect of all four lifestyle elements makes the transformative difference.

- **Nutrition:** Enjoy nourishingly delicious meals and discover friendly ways to prepare them at home.

- **Stress Management:** Learn a range of relaxation techniques, release stress, and react in healthier ways.

- **Fitness:** Experience the vitality that comes from moderate daily activity.

- **Love and Support:** Give and receive emotional support to help unlock the healing power of the community.

The Proven Lifestyle

When we become more aware of how much our choices in diet and lifestyle affect us—for better and for worse—then we can make different ones. When you make healthy choices, you feel better quickly. This allows us to connect the dots between what we do and how we feel. Feeling so much better, so quickly, reframes the reason for changing from fear of dying to joy of living.

People often think that advances in medicine have to be a new drug, a new laser, or a surgical intervention to be powerful—something really high-tech and expensive. They often have a hard time believing that the simple choices that we make in our lives each day—what we eat, how we respond to stress, whether or not we smoke, how much we exercise, and the quality of our relationships—can make such a powerful difference in our health, our well-being, and our survival, but they often do. Awareness is the first step in healing. When we become more aware of how powerfully our choices in diet and lifestyle affect us—for better and for worse—then we can make different ones. It's like connecting the dots between what we do and how we feel.

Part of the value of science is to raise our awareness by helping us to understand the powerful effects of the diet and lifestyle choices we make each day—and how changing these may significantly, sometimes dramatically, improve our health and well-being. In many cases, these improvements may occur much more quickly than people had once believed possible.

The Research

Dr. Ornish's 37 years of research have scientifically proven that the integrative lifestyle changes he recommends can:

- Improve chronic conditions – such as heart disease, diabetes, and prostate cancer.

- Change gene expression, turning on health-promoting genes and turning off disease-promoting genes.

- Lengthen telomeres — the ends of chromosomes — which begin to reverse aging on a cellular level.

The Benefits

- Feel more energy.
- Improve your quality of life.
- Lower your chances of needing surgery.
- Reduce your risk of a heart-related event.
- Anticipate and manage stress effectively.
- With your doctor's guidance, reduce or discontinue many and sometimes all medications.

The *Ornish Lifestyle Medicine* Program

In the East, where I hail from originally, there is a saying about life and learning: When the student is ready, the teacher appears! When I joined this nine-week program, the teacher appeared; not just one, but many who work as a team to educate, train, and coach the new group of so-called cohorts.

The Ornish Program Team at The Hunterdon Medical Center is composed of a Rehab. Program Director, Registered Nurses, Exercise Physiologists, Registered Dietitian Nutritionists, Stress Management Specialists, Executive Chef, and Administration and Housekeeping Staff. Most of them are trained by the Ornish Organization in the methodology underlying the four aspects: nutrition, stress management, fitness, and love and support. The program directors are cardiologists from the Hunterdon Cardiovascular Associates Group, and the program is sponsored by them. Each participant's cardiologist/physician is regularly updated with the progress report of their patient—thus making him/her a part of the team as well. This is what I may refer to as the "dream team" of competent professionals dedicated to the health and well-being of needy patients. I could not have asked for a better solution to attempt and reverse my heart disease. I express my gratitude to these noble souls. Now, the rest was up to me!

The nine-week, 72-hour program, is scheduled as follows: two days a week, for four hours a day, the cohorts (all patients enrolled in one class) go through these segments: One hour of moderate aerobic exercises, followed by one hour of facilitated open discussion of feelings and challenges, thus laying the foundation for Ornish alumni to continue their support relationship beyond the program. This is followed by one hour of stress management practice, concluding with one hour of eating a plant-based-Ornish-approved lunch menu prepared by the executive chef. During lunch, the dietitian explains the menu, its ingredients, and sources to buy from. The dietitian also provides education in how to read food product labels to be wise about eating healthy choices and eliminating processed food. The participants are encouraged to have their family member/spouse/partner participate in the lunch and educational presentations. (This is a smart thing to do because, for the participant, it would be hard to explain what, why, and how of the Ornish approach when they would go home. This eases the challenges of their transition.)

By learning and practicing the four aspects of the Ornish methodology, I had noticed that in addition to the practice becoming a habit; I was getting transformed in new ways about my choices of foods. My wife has been cooking for me for about one-half century, with just about no interest on my part to learn to cook. The ideas of the Ornish

Program's acceptable food and their preparation sparked my interest in learning to cook myself. My wife coached me in the basics of how to cut onions, for example, and how to use Indian spices—as I mostly eat Indian foods. Yes, cutting onions, some people may laugh at this! I bought an Instant Pot, the comprehensive, easy-to-use pressure cooker. And bravo, I had started to enjoy cooking plant-based foods. Even my wife started to like some of my cooking. In conjunction with the stress management aspect, I found preparing and cooking to be therapeutic.

The second interesting by-product of this program was me starting to do food shopping. The Ornish Reversal Program provided us with reference cards to carry for shopping and cooking choices. Again, my wife shopped for food always. With the Ornish Guidelines Cards in hand, I started to read labels on food products in the supermarket. I found it remarkably interesting and started to enjoy it. Reading food labels was an eye-opening experience. Many packaged products have so many processed ingredients that one can't even pronounce their names, never mind understanding what these alien items are. My wife got tired of me spending so much time reading labels on the products while grocery shopping that I decided to go shopping on my own. I had a new hobby. If I see a label and don't understand the ingredients' names and they don't complement my new diet —I quickly put those back on the shelf.

This reminds me of a story: In a Punjab village, once, a visitor came and needed to look up the meaning of a rather difficult word in his language. He asked an elder: "Is there a lughat in the village which I may use?" (the Urdu language word for dictionary is lughat). "Why do you need it?" asked the elder. "I need to look up the meaning of a challenging word," said the visitor. The elder replied: "In our village, we only speak the words that we all understand, and therefore don't need a lughat."

This has become my new mantra for reading food labels! If I don't understand, I put an item back and don't plan to eat it again. Meal planning has become enjoyable. Through positive feedback, i.e., I've lost weight, insulin demand has decreased, the motivation to continue is quite natural. While reading food labels and cooking may be trivial for many, these have been a step-change in my health transformation journey.

The Ornish Program also includes access to a comprehensive library of all the supporting tools, techniques, and relevant literature. This access remains available even after graduation from the nine-week course. In addition, daily eating logs are provided on the website for tracking progress. These are reviewed by the dietitian. It is worth noting that there are new and updated Nutrition Facts Labels for food. It is good to be aware of the labels' information. The details are available on the FDA's website, https://bit.ly/3hnAF0x.

FDA Nutrition Facts Label

The US Food and Drug Administration (FDA) has updated the Nutrition Facts label on packaged foods and drinks. The FDA requires changes to the Nutrition Facts label based on updated scientific information, new nutrition research, and input from the public. This is the first major update to the label in over 20 years. The label's refreshed design and updated information will make it easier for you to make informed food choices that contribute to lifelong healthy eating habits.

Nutrition Facts

8 servings per container
Serving size   **2/3 cup (55g)**

Amount per serving
Calories   **230**

% Daily Value*

Total Fat 8g	**10%**
Saturated Fat 1g	**5%**
Trans Fat 0g	
Cholesterol 0mg	**0%**
Sodium 160mg	**7%**
Total Carbohydrate 37g	**13%**
Dietary Fiber 4g	**14%**
Total Sugars 12g	
Includes 10g Added Sugars	**20%**
Protein 3g	
Vitamin D 2mcg	10%
Calcium 260mg	20%
Iron 8mg	45%
Potassium 235mg	6%

* The % Daily Value (DV) tells you how much a nutrient in a serving of food contributes to a daily diet. 2,000 calories a day is used for general nutrition advice.

1. The serving size now appears in larger, bold font and some serving sizes have been updated.

2. Calories are now displayed in larger, bolder font.

3. Daily Values have been updated.

4. Added sugars, vitamin D, and potassium are now listed. Manufacturers must declare the amount in addition to percent Daily Value for vitamins and minerals.

Figure 5.3 FDA Nutrition Facts Label

1: **Serving Sizes Get Real**. Servings per container and serving size information appear in large, bold font. Serving sizes have also been updated to reflect better the amount people typically eat and drink today. Note: The serving size is not a recommendation of how much to eat.

2: **Calories Go Big**. Calories are now in larger and bolder font to make the information easier to find and use.

3: **The Lows and Highs of % Daily Value**. The percent Daily Value (%DV) shows how much of a nutrient in a serving of food contributes to a total daily diet.

4. **Nutrients.** The Updated List. Based on research, some information is no longer required on the label, e.g., Calories from Fat, and Vitamins A and C; Some information has been added, such as Added Sugars, Vitamin D and Potassium.

Back to Ornish Methodology. In the Ornish Lifestyle Medicine program, I had learned the proposed food label ingredients and preparation guideline which was immensely helpful as a quick reference cheat sheet for shopping or for cooking at home.

"**Acceptable** food label ingredients. Fat sources (mainly unsaturated)

Canola Oil, Monoglycerides, Diglycerides, Nut Oils (except coconut), Seed Oils. Soybean Oil, Nuts and Seeds,

Corn oil, Lectin, Olive Oil, Safflower Oil. (Limit low-fat foods to less than or equal to three servings/day.)

Unacceptable food label ingredients. Fat sources (mainly saturated)

Butter, Chicken Fat, Coconut Oil, Cream, Egg Yolks, Hydrogenated Oils, Beef Fat/Tallow, Low/Whole Fat Milk Products, Margarine, Palm/Palm Kernel Oil, Shortening, Lard.

Preparation: Vegetarian: No meat, poultry, fish, seafood, egg yolks, or low-fat dairy products. Nonfat dairy and egg whites are allowed in limited amounts. Fat-Free: No added oil, butter, or margarine. No nuts, seeds, avocado, or coconut. May use small amounts of non-stick spray.

There is even a **Chef Card** provided in the program that one can take to restaurants and show to chefs so that they may be able to accommodate one's dietary requirements.

Ornish Reversal Program Education Included:

Introduction to stress management, nutrition, and fitness, tracking for success, listening with empathy, meal planning, stress toolkit, plant-based nutrition, cooking essentials, and mindful-presence-eating.

The structure of the nine-week program enables a new life approach to become a habit. In stress management, there are several techniques, which include yoga, stretching, and deep relaxation. I practice this therapy almost daily now. My most favorite is the deep relaxation posture, described in the following article in *Ornish Living Newsletter* on the Ornish website.

To the fitness program, I have added some additional exercises that include visualization, yoga, Qigong and Tai Chi postures. Under the Love and Support, I have added my own concept called taking daily "Vitamin F." As other daily supplements, this is a reminder to call family and friends and stay connected.

Finding Calm by Turning Upside Down, by Susi Amendola, Stress Management Specialist. Article included here with the permission of Ornish Organization.

Sigh…daily life is stressful. Whether it's the mounting pressures of work, navigating family and relationships, or the chaos and turmoil we feel when we turn on the news, it all has an effect on our health and well-being. The shoulder stand is a classic inversion that lets the nervous system and heart power down.

Chronic stress takes its toll on the body by raising stress hormones like adrenaline and cortisol. Cortisol increases sugars (glucose) in the bloodstream while adrenaline increases your heart rate, elevates your blood pressure, and boosts energy so you can prepare to fight or flee. These stress hormones interfere with the peaceful internal environment we need to cultivate for optimal health. For this reason, practicing some stress management will help to stay balanced and calm in the midst of everyday life.

The Queen of Yoga Postures. There are many techniques and practices from which to choose in order to calm down. Modified shoulder stand, however, is one of the most powerful as well as my personal favorite for restoring overall health and well-being. It's a classic inversion that lets the nervous system and heart power down. It is considered the queen of yoga postures because of its overall impact on the body and mind.

How Shoulder Stand is Done and Why it's Helpful: a) Lying on the floor, place one-bed pillow under the back of the pelvis. b) Then, place both legs up on the seat of a chair. Try to support the calves up through the back of the knees. C) Now, place a second bed pillow under the back of the head, so the chin is slightly tucked downward. D) Let yourself relax and breathe. E) Stay in this position for 3-15 mins at a time.

The Effect of Shoulder Stand. When the legs are elevated, the blood from the legs starts to drain back toward the pelvis and lower back. This provides some venous return and reduces the load on the veins of the legs. It also pools the blood in the abdomen so that the low back is bathed with a fresh supply of blood. Additionally, it releases the lumbar curve and takes the strain off the low back by releasing any tensions you may have stored there.

With the pillow under the buttocks, the pooling blood in the abdomen is then lifted toward the heart, delivering additional blood flow to the heart and lungs. This blood is then carried to the neck. Since there is a pillow under the head, the chin is tucked down, so there is a second pooling of blood in the area of the thyroid gland and the carotid arteries. The thyroid is the master gland responsible for controlling metabolism.

The carotid arteries are the receptors that tell the brain that the heart has enough blood, and it doesn't need to pump so hard. <u>So, in turn, heart rate and blood pressure both go down.</u> While the initial inclination is for the blood pressure to rise when we are upside down, it may rise momentarily. In a few minutes, however, the heart rate lowers, and the body adjusts to the mild inversion. The blood pressure also comes down, thereby improving blood pressure variability as well.

The Key to the Most Benefit. The key is that the pillow lifts the buttocks, and the second pillow tucks the chin down so the blood pools in the abdomen and then the neck. <u>This is why it is often referred to as the pose of two waterfalls. One waterfall of blood and energy extends from the legs to the abdomen and one from the abdomen to the neck.</u>

Lying in this position also drains the lymph. The lymphatic system is not a pumped system, so there is additional support given to it when we rest the legs up on the chair. The brain and the spinal cord form the control center known as the central nervous system. The cervical (neck) nerves control sensations in *the body and breathing. When the neck is tucked down, it sends a message through those nerves to rest the nervous system.*

Taking time to rest in this deeply restorative mild inversion posture provides maximum benefits in managing the ups and downs of our ordinary lives. It teaches us how to remain calm when everything is turned upside down. Try it and see. Your body may just thank you for the help.

Consider Seated Chair Version for These Conditions. *You may want to consult your doctor about this alternate shoulder stand if you have any of the following: Menstruation, GERD (Reflux), and Hiatal Hernia, Significant cervical/spinal arthritis, Labile Hypertension, Vagal Syncope, Significant Carotid Stenosis, History of Stroke, Retinopathy, Retinal Hemorrhage, Detached Retina, Glaucoma. (Source: https://www.ornish.com/ornish-living/).*

Figure 5.4 shows a diagram of the Shoulder Stand. This has become my favorite tool, which I prefer to call **Deep Relaxation**. First, I perform breath and stretch exercises followed by deep relaxation. I keep my room dark; place my legs on a chair with a pillow on top, one pillow under my buttocks and one under my head. I cover myself with a blanket for warmth. I play light meditation music on my mobile phone.

Within four to five minutes of this posture, as I perform a meditation mantra in my mind, I suddenly get a sensation of a slow-down-trigger in the body. It is metaphorically like when a car has its engine racing, and we may change the gear to neutral, the engine starts to what is called idling. Immediately thereafter, my body and mind go into a relaxed stage…a sort of sleep but not as deeply asleep as I have when I lie in my bed. I may stay in this mode from one-half hour to an hour. When I get up, I am more alert and energetic than if I would be lying in bed. It is the kind of sleep where you are asleep but are aware that you are sleeping. As the article above states, I believe the heart suddenly goes into "idling" and has time to relax and work less hard.

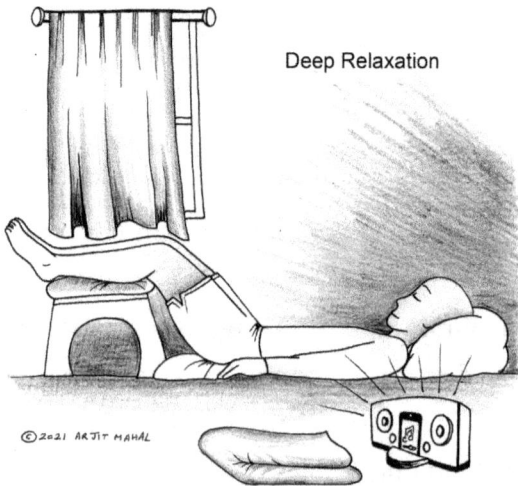

Figure 5.4 Deep Relaxation

Ornish Program Discharge Report October 2020

Throughout the program, the progress of the participants is very closely monitored, and periodic reports are sent to one's sponsoring cardiologist; at the end, a comprehensive report is prepared and shared. In addition to the Anthropometrics (the study of human body measurements) and blood work, the progress of the participant in each of the four segments of the program is detailed. Here are some key data points of my nine-week participation. The numbers "speak" for themselves.

Measure	Initial Assessment	Discharge Assessment	Difference
Anthropometrics			
Height (in &cm)	68.5/173.99	68.5/173.99	None
Weight (lbs/kg)	187.6/85.27	172.5/78.41	-15.1/-6.86
BMI (Body Mass Index)	28.11	25.84	-2.27
Waist (Inches)	41.5	39	-2.5
Hip (Inches)	42.5	38	-4.5
Waist/Hip Ratio	0.98	1.03	+ 0.05
Blood Pressure			
Resting SBP	134	118	-16
Resting DBP	72	60	-12
Functional Capacity			
METS	4.2	2.5	-1.7
Blood Work			
Total Cholesterol	157	98	-59
LDL	90	42	-48
HDL	38	34	-4 (genetically low)
Triglycerides	203	136	-67
Chol/HDL Ratio	4.13	2.9	-1.23
HgbA1c	6.8 (With 4 times insulin)	7.1 (With 1-time low dose)	+0.3
Hs-CRP	Not available	0.6	In Range

Table 5.3 Ornish Program Discharge Report

Note: This does not mean that I don't take any medication for my heart. I continue to take medications of CHD protocol since I have stents installed, and certain vitals must be kept in check. These include aspirin and statin regimen. Medication details are out of the scope of this book.

Table Legend:[12]

METS stands for metabolic equivalence. It is a physiologic measurement of how much energy your body expends on exertion relative to the mass of that person. It is defined as the amount of oxygen consumed.

Waist/Hip Ratio and waist circumference are reliable and simple tools to measure abdominal obesity, and we know that if we have a greater circumference around our waist than hips, we are more predisposed to cardiovascular disease and diabetes with a higher risk of morbidity and mortality. BMI (body mass index) measures body size and composition and provides additional information regarding being underweight and overweight. The goal for W/H ratio for males is.0.9 or less (according to WHO)...in both men and women, a WHR of 1.0 or higher increases the risk for heart disease.

----

[12] Definitions Source: Hunterdon Cardiac Rehab Staff.

C-Peptide Test

An additional test was done separately on October 5, 2020, to determine whether my pancreas was producing more insulin as compared to a test done on June 1, 2020. The result in Table 5.4 shown the improvement, which I attribute to my overall effort of health transformation. It shows that my pancreas had started to make more insulin. Of course, the fact remained that my insulin antibodies are attacking it. A simple conceptual diagram in Figure 5.5 Insulin & Partners shows the origin of insulin, C-peptide, and glucagon. Insulin and C-Peptide are produced by Beta Cells, and Glucagon is produced by the Alpha Cells.

June 1, 2020	October 5, 2020	Reference Range
1.42	2.03	0.80-3.85 ng/mL.

Table 5.4 C-Peptide Test Result Oct. 2020.

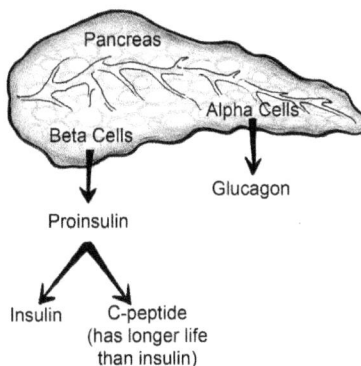

Figure 5.5 Insulin and Partners

After the nine-week Ornish Lifestyle Medicine Program, and upon our graduation, as a gesture of our gratitude, we, the cohorts, made the following presentation to honor the entire team by presenting a plaque to the experts who had trained and coached us.

We, the Cohorts Class Members, express our gratitude to the Cardiac Rehab Staff for providing us education, practice, guidance, and encouragement in all four aspects of the Ornish Undo It! Program. The Ornish Methodology is a step-by-step approach designed to incrementally enable us to manage our heart healing and health with effective tools and techniques—which we believe will be a part of our life-long persona in nutrition, fitness, stress, and support. Notwithstanding our gratefulness to the Hunterdon Medical Center for their dedication to our cause, we are indebted to the entire Ornish Program Team:

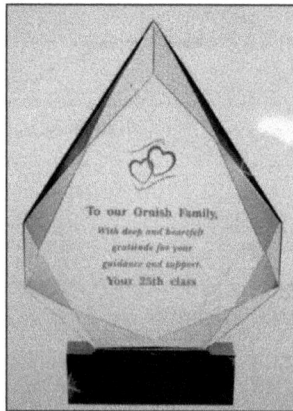

Figure 5.6 Gratitude Plaque

Program Director, Registered Nurses, Exercise Physiologists, Registered Dietitian Nutritionists, Stress Management Specialists, Executive Chef, and Administration and House Keeping Staff. In these three words, we can describe the entire team: COMPETENT CARING COMPASSIONATE. (The plaque reads: To our Ornish Family: With deep and heartfelt gratitude for your guidance and support. Your 25th class.)

While I cannot do anything about the grafts and stents in my heart, I can eliminate or minimize the contributing factors that cause and propagate coronary artery disease. Doing nothing would be irresponsible for me.

This sums up all about my experience with the *Ornish Lifestyle Undo It! Program.*

This has been my next major step in my health transformation journey.

CHAPTER 6

Weight

> We do not get fat because we overeat. We overeat because we get fat.
>
> **Gary Taubes, in his book:**
> *Why We Get Fat: And What to Do About It*

All my life, I could say I was on the chubby side, not obese, but rather overweight per the standard BMI Scale. For many years I had my weight fluctuating between 170 and 175 pounds, until I was put on insulin. My naturopath doctor, Dr. Francis Cinelli, who has 60 some years of experience, told me once that many years ago, when a patient wanted to increase his/her weight, it was a standard practice to prescribe insulin. When I started to take insulin a couple of years ago, my weight jumped from 170 to 190 pounds—no matter how much I dieted or exercised. Upon learning of a book by Dr. Jason Fung, I understood why insulin is the culprit. It is a vicious cycle of some diabetes medications such as insulin: take medication, increase in weight, increase insulin, more increase in weight. The physicians just say well, you can expect insulin to increase weight!

By being on a plant-based diet and practicing Ornish Lifestyle Medicine, I had started to lose weight—as a by-product of my effort. Let us look at weight measures and what that may mean. One measure is BMI to determine where one stands in terms of a standard for an adult (it may differ for men versus women and children).

According to the CDC (Center for Disease Control and Prevention), BMI is a person's weight in kilograms divided by the square of height in meters. BMI is an inexpensive and easy screening method for weight category— underweight, healthy weight, overweight, and obesity. BMI does not measure body fat directly, but BMI is moderately correlated with more direct measures of body fat. Furthermore, BMI appears to be strongly correlated with various metabolic and disease outcomes, as are these more direct measures of body fatness.

How is BMI calculated? BMI is calculated the same way for both adults and children. The body mass index formula is a simple calculation that takes into account your weight and height:

```
The imperial BMI formula = Weight
(Pounds) x 703 ÷ Height (Inches²)

The metric BMI formula = Weight
(Kilograms) ÷ Height (Meters²).
```

```
My own BMI now is: 160 x 703 =
112480. Divide it by 4624 (my
height is 68 inches square). So,
112480 divided by 4624 = 24 BMI.
```

According to the standards table below, I am now in the healthy/normal weight category. Before I had started my health transformation, my BMI was 28, so I was in the overweight category. There are numerous websites which have quick calculators for BMI, including the National Heart, Lung & Blood Institute: BMI Calculation, https://bit.ly/3y4D0Ek. The standard weight status categories associated with BMI are shown in Figure 6.1.

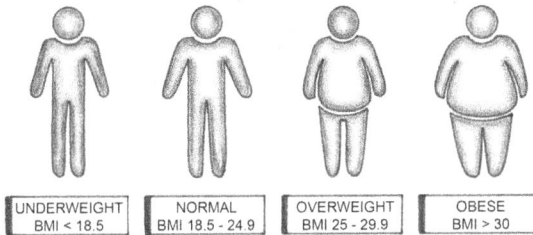

UNDERWEIGHT	NORMAL	OVERWEIGHT	OBESE
BMI < 18.5	BMI 18.5 - 24.9	BMI 25 - 29.9	BMI > 30

© 2021 ARJIT MAHAL

Figure 6.1 BMI Conceptual View

At 175 pounds before starting insulin, my BMI was 26.2. So I was in the overweight category. After a couple of years on the insulin medication, my weight rose to over 190 pounds, and my BMI was 28.9. Not obese yet, but it was heading in that direction. *What do I do?* The answer was addressed by Dr. Jason Fung in his book: *The Obesity Code, Unlocking the Secrets of Weight Loss* (Greystone Books)

Pages 73-76. Figure 6.2 contains the author's conceptual view of the underlying biological processes inspired by Dr. Fung's statements on obesity and the underlying biological processes. The process steps are pathway numbers for reference.

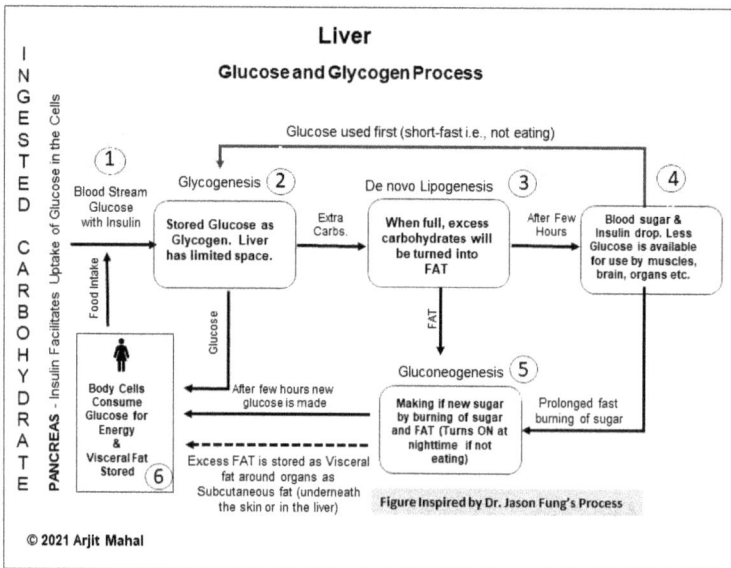

Figure 6.2 Liver, Glucose & Glycogen Process

When we eat (Step 1), except for the dietary fiber, the food is broken down in our stomach into amino acids, fatty acids, and sugar. Blood sugar stimulates the pancreas to release insulin into the bloodstream. When more glucose is created than needed by the body, it is stored in the liver as glycogen (Step 2). Glycogen functions as a form of energy reserve stored primarily in the cells of the liver and skeletal muscle for later use. This process is called Glycogenesis, being the origin or beginning of something new. Thus, the process of Glycogenesis is stimulated by the hormone insulin.

The extra dietary carbohydrates are converted into fat by a process called De novo Lipogenesis, meaning the making of new fat (Step 3). In between the meals, after a few hours of not eating, the blood glucose concentration drops, and the liver starts to convert stored glycogen into glucose for energy for the body's organs— Gluconeogenesis, the reverse of Glycogenesis occurs. (Steps 4 & 5).

During a short-term fast, your body has enough glycogen available to function. During a prolonged fast, your body can make new glucose from its fat stores…We eat, insulin goes up, and we store energy as glycogen and fat…We fast, insulin goes down, and we use our stored energy…

Dr. Fung

For me, understanding this glucose and glycogen process was the beginning of the awareness in terms of the balance needed for eating, fasting, and managing my weight better. Of course, there are many other complex biological/neurological processes that include calories in and calories out, hormonal activities to regulate hunger and body set weight, insulin resistance in the case of my type 2 diabetes condition, etc. High insulin levels in the bloodstream and the body's cells not being able to absorb glucose for energy is called insulin resistance.

As I was on an insulin regimen to manage my blood glucose numbers, I needed more insulin to process the glucose in the bloodstream when I ate more than I should have eaten. Therefore, due to insulin resistance, I realized that the glucose and insulin in my bloodstream were backing up like a traffic jam in my tunnel, resulting in more insulin resistance by the cells and, of course, more weight gain. This persistence of high insulin level is called hyperinsulinemia (hyperinsulinemia means that the amount of insulin in your blood is higher than what is considered normal). So, the same insulin that helps manage diabetes can also the potential cause of type 2 diabetes. Dr. Jason Fung refers to this dilemma as "Diabesity, the "new science of diabetes", and further states that "We have seen the enemy, and it is ourselves."

This is the example of what the father of toxicology, Paracelsus, stated in the sixteenth century: The dose makes the poison; anything can be harmful in excessive amounts, even if it is typically considered beneficial. Just as insulin and other medications for managing diabetes could have a similar effect, I must find a way to reduce or eliminate insulin intake. It seemed logical that if I could "control" my diet and reduce my weight, I may be able to tackle "diabesity", the interplay of diabetes and obesity—feeding off each other. While I did not fall in the classification of obese, per the BMI Index, the above information was enough for me to get motivated to start some basic steps in my health transformation. I never explored diets such as calorie counting and lowering carbohydrates, with names such as the Atkins Diet and Paleo Diet, because I do not like to measure and track calories.

Among his other recommendations, I was particularly impressed by Dr. Fung's suggestion of fasting as a process to manage the insulin imbalance. Dr. Fung suggests that fasting is an ancient remedy practiced by many cultures and religions for centuries. So rather than searching for some exotic diet miracle to break insulin resistance, why not try this ancient healing tradition? (See Chapter 8. Fasting.)

In my health transformation journey, including weight reduction, these three things made all the difference:

- Plant-Based-Diet
- Fasting
- Body and Mind Balance (Ornish Lifestyle Medicine).

Practicing the above disciplines over time, my weight loss progress was natural. And it reduced drug intake to very minimal levels on ad hoc basis. Weight loss from over 190 pounds to 160 pounds, thirty pounds loss, resulted in my blood work numbers being the best I can remember. My cholesterol profile became normal, and my diabetes Type 2 insulin resistance became less. Overall, I started to feel better and have positive energy in my body and mind.

I am also a type 1.5 diabetic, meaning that my natural insulin is attacked by insulin autoantibodies and therefore causes insulin deficiency. (Ironically, this is the opposite of the insulin resistance issue!) I must find out how to treat that condition which I have been told does not have an easy solution. That said, I am working with one my physicians and a special laboratory CYREX Laboratories in Arizona, USA (www.cyresLabs.com), to first understand the condition and then determine some course of corrective action—if possible. My blood plasma was sent to the laboratory for testing, the result came back stating that I have "Array 6" and the specific technical data was reported under the title, "Diabetes Autoimmune Reactivity Screen." The laboratory does not provide any prescriptive solution, but their scientists provide consultation to the physicians with possible options. As a result of this consultation, my physician has put me on a natural healing protocol that includes supplements and special compounds. Even if there may not be a cure, I am hoping for an improvement in my condition. I don't give up easily! This may be a story for another time.

When the diet is wrong medicine is of no use, when the diet is correct medicine is of no need.

An Ayurvedic proverb

CHAPTER 7

Nutrition

There are not more than five cardinal tastes (sour, acrid, salt, sweet, bitter), yet combinations of them yield more flavors than can ever be tasted.

Sun Tzu (544 BC-496 BC)

I am not a trained expert in nutrition, so what I am sharing in this book is my personal and practical experience—which has worked for me. However, I can write about some of the foods I have been eating that helped my transformation for better health and well-being. For this, I am uniquely qualified. Thus, this is the scope of this chapter: my own nutrition and food approach. As in any journey, before starting, one must look at maps, routes, terrains, and possibilities—to ensure the successful arrival at the destination. In this context, I mean identifying philosophy and principle for self "Journey." I am not providing any deep-dive research, nor do I intend to provide proof of my deductions and ideas.

The reader may take away what makes sense to them, or at minimum, they may get inspired to create their own framework of nutrition and foods—based on their individual needs. Recipes and such are not in the scope of this book. I have included my generic recipe template for cooking what I have learned and enjoy eating. In addition, there are a few experimental recipes for beginners who may want to be on a plant-based diet and want to learn cooking.

Mayo Clinic Foundation for Medical Education and Research, in its publication *The Recipe for Healthy Digestion, Steps for Living, Eating and Staying Active*, has this to say:

"Good health and healthy gut go hand in hand. Digestion is one of the critical functions your body must perform to survive and thrive. The food you eat provides necessary nutrients that supply your cells with sustenance and energy so your body can develop, repair and maintain itself...the digestion process breaks down food into smaller components and change it chemically so nutrients can be extracted and absorbed into your bloodstream (while the remainder is eliminated as waste)."

This above publication further states: "What you put on your plate has a lot to do with your digestion. But it's not only what you eat that's important. How much you eat and how you eat— relaxed or hurried, focused or distracted—also play key roles. Your daily food choices and eating habits go a long way toward keeping your digestive system strong and healthy...If you can stick with these changes, gradually, they become habits. Those habits, in turn, become a routine, and eventually, that routine becomes your new lifestyle. The benefits are many. In addition to improving your digestive health, healthier habits can reduce your risk of disease and help you look and feel your best."

Natural Laws of Nutrition – My Adopted Principles

Based on my learnings and commonsense, I have developed my own set of guiding principles. These have worked for me with success.

Eat foods in a natural and unaltered state. This means eat what is least touched by humans in terms of processed food. Some food corporations take out nutrients from natural products then put them back with more stuff for taste or for shelf life.

Eat when hungry. The concept of timing for three meals and such is probably an invention of the industrial age. Our ancient ancestors did not have clocks to set their time, other than the cycle of the day and night. The animals eat when they are hungry. It's ok to be hungry; you'll appreciate the next meal even more.

Eat human "sense" foods. Our subconscious tells us whether the food is good for us or not. But our mind gets tempted to eat because much of the processed food industry has "designed" the eatables to fool our five senses. Listen to your subconscious and try to harness the mind.

Respect Life-Sustaining Air, Water, Earth. Guru Nanak had said *"pavan guroo paanee pitaa maataa dharat mahat; divas raat du-ay daa-ee daa-i-aa khaylai sagal jagat."* Air is the Guru (a teacher who gives us life's light), Water is the Father, and Earth is the Great Mother of all; Day and night are the two nurses, in whose lap all the world is at play."

Laws of Eating I Follow

Mindful Presence and Eating

Focus on here and now. First, express gratitude, think of all the farmers who grew/produced your food, and all those who supported the supply chain. <u>Avoid other distractions when eating</u>. (*Source: Mind & Body. Mayo Clinic Women's Health Science, January 2011).*

Eknath Easwaran was an Indian-born spiritual teacher who had migrated to America from India. He used to tell the story of when he was a child. He was fond of eating *Idli* (rice cakes). He was also fond of reading. So, he would be reading the book holding in one hand and eating *Idlis,* one after the other, from his plate. His grandmother lectured him and said, "Son, if you eat and read at the same time, you don't savor the food; and besides, your subconscious is split...you won't comprehend what you are reading. Do only one thing at a time."

Plant-Based Food – *"Buddha Bowl"*

I don't like to be called a vegan. I prefer to say that I eat Mother-Earth-Foods that grow under the earth and above the earth. I try to have multicolor raw vegetables along with pickles, pickled pearl onions, pickled sushi ginger, sauerkraut, edamame (protein, I have not been able to get used to Tofu yet). This approach reduces my carbon footprint on earth (my little effort). Buddha Bowls, the trendy name, is given to colorful bowls of vegetables, grains, proteins, and other healthy foods. Savoring each of the items is a pleasure—which I had never experienced before.

Low Glycemic Index (GI) Foods

Patrick J. Skerrett, Former Executive Editor, *Harvard Health, explains in simple terms in his article: Use a glycemic index to help control blood sugar (August 13, 2012).*

"Picture an old-fashioned roller coaster with plenty of ups and downs. That's what your blood sugar and insulin levels look like over the course of a day. The highs that follow meals and snacks drop to lows later on. Learning to eat in a way that makes your blood sugar levels look more like a kiddie coaster with gentle ups and downs than a strap-'em-in, hang-on-tight ride with steep climbs and breathtaking drops can make a difference to your health. How can you do this? A tool called the glycemic index (GI) can help. It rates carbohydrate-containing foods by how much they boost blood sugar (blood glucose). As someone with diabetes, I use the glycemic index as one strategy to keep my blood sugar under control. And there may be other benefits—low glycemic index diets have been linked to reduced risks for cancer, heart disease, and other conditions."

The University of Sydney, Australia, maintains an extensive database of GI. This can be used as a guide for planning and creating eating habits at http://www.glycemicindex.com/about.php. On their website, relevant to diabetes, I found the following information useful—for my purpose.

"When we consume carb-rich foods, our bodies convert their sugars and starches to glucose, but it converts them at very different rates. Some foods break down quickly during digestion, and the glucose in the bloodstream increases rapidly; others break down slowly, and the glucose is released gradually into the blood. And, of course, there are moderates. The GI is a numerical ranking that provides a good indication of how fast the body will digest, absorb, and metabolize carb foods that have been tested following the international standard. But the GI is only part of the story. It can only measure carb-containing foods, and it's not always proportional to the insulin response to a food. When our blood glucose levels rise, our pancreas releases insulin (a hormone) that drives the glucose out of our bloodstream and into our body's cells where our body can use it as an immediate source of energy or store it as glycogen."

At this stage, I find that we must keep in mind, sometimes a bit confusing difference between "insulin resistance" and "insulin sensitivity." The University's website gives a clear explanation:

"You are what's called 'insulin sensitive'—a good thing—if you require relatively little insulin to process your BGLs (blood glucose levels). On the other hand, if your body needs to secrete a lot of insulin into the blood, you have "insulin resistance". We sometimes describe it as your body being "partially deaf" to insulin. Think of it like this: just as we may shout to make a deaf person hear, the body needs to make more insulin to drive glucose where it's supposed to go. So, moving glucose from the blood into cells necessitates the release of large amounts of insulin...How can you optimize your insulin sensitivity and decrease insulin levels over the whole day? A healthy low GI diet plus physical activity are the most powerful ways to do this, as numerous studies have shown...."

Note: University of Sydney's GI News of March 2021 states: The vast majority of published GI values are of Western origin, notably European, Australian, and North American. We know that GI values are altered by the degree of cooking and processing, and this will vary from country to country. Now they have new data on South Asian Food Glycemic Index, https://ginews.blogspot.com/.

Below is one more useful tip from the University of Sydney's website, which helped me with an a-ha moment, the benefit of vinegar in managing diabetes.

"...One reason many fermented foods are beneficial to health is the production of organic acids such as lactic acid and acetic acid (the same acid as in **vinegar**). These are by-products of the fermentation process when the bacteria/yeast metabolizes carbohydrates (sugars and starches) in the food or drink. These organic acids not only add distinctive flavors to the food or drink; they also lower the pH (a measure of acidity and alkalinity of a solution), making it difficult for harmful microorganisms to grow. In our stomachs, they slow down a food's rate of emptying into the intestine, which in turn slows the rate of digestion and absorption of the food's carbohydrates into the bloodstream, lowering the overall GI...."

No Animal Foods or Products—No Oils/Fats

Use a spray of olive oil or canola oil, just to sauté the cooked food such as lentils, beans. Even vegetable stock can be used to lightly sauté foods.

Eat Wisely

Eat when hungry. When you are about 80% full, push the plate away (and, of course, don't fill the plate to avoid wastage). Don't go for seconds. The stomach may be full, but the mind may be tempting you (be aware). After putting food in the mouth, put the fork or spoon down. This slows down the risk of gobbling food, and more saliva will be mixed in with food to help in digestion.

Drink Food and Eat Water

This means to chew the solid food to the point that it becomes liquid, and drink water as if you are eating, i.e., one sip at a time (not gulp down). My grandfather used to advise: "The reason we have 32 teeth is that nature wants us to chew a bite of food 32 times." On drinking water. Unlike most of the East, in the West, particularly the United States, people drink cold water from the refrigerator and even put ice in it. I have not done enough reading of Ayurvedic philosophy to understand why cold water is not good for the body. Maybe our microbiome ecosystem does not welcome this onslaught of cold in a warm environment inside our body! I prefer to drink water at room temperature and even make it a bit warmer when eating with food. One should do their own due diligence.

Fasting has been around from the beginning of human history. Many cultures and religions around the globe promote fasting. Sometimes the fasting is tied to social or religious ceremonies to ensure it is done as a practice and habit.

In his book, *The Obesity Code,* Dr. Jason Fung states: "...The ancient Greeks believed that medical treatment could be discovered by observing nature. Humans, like most animals, do not eat when they become sick...The ancient Greeks also believed that fasting improved cognitive abilities...As a healing tradition, fasting has a long history. Hippocrates of Kos (c.460-c.370 BC) is widely considered the father of modern medicine. Among the treatment that he prescribed and championed were the practice of fasting and the consumption of apple cider vinegar. Hippocrates wrote, "To eat when you are sick is to feed your illness."

Greek writer and historian Plutarch (c. AD 46-c. AD 120) also echoed these sentiments. He wrote, "Instead of using medicine better, fast today." Plato and his student Aristotle were also staunch supporters of fasting. Other intellectual giants were also great proponents of fasting.

Paracelsus (1493-1541), the founder of toxicology and one of the three fathers of modern western medicine (along with Hippocrates and Galen), wrote, *Fasting is the greatest remedy—the physician within.* Benjamin Franklin (1706-1790), one of America's founding fathers and renowned for wide knowledge, once wrote of fasting, "The best of all medicines is resting and fasting."

In the chapter on fasting, I go into detail on my own positive experience.

Brain Dump of Thoughts And Ideas

Humans and Animals

Human ancestors are known to be "hunter-gatherers." In my opinion, it should be "gatherer hunters." It is highly likely that they ate Mother Earth Foods prior to meats. It was only when they learned how to harness fire that they would have started cooking meat (can't eat raw meat). Human jaws and teeth are designed for chewing vegetation – not meat (that is what nature intended).

The human digestive system/intestines are longer than that of carnivores. It is designed to digest slowly, as we don't have enzymes that can dissolve meat easily. Food may stay for two days in the system without harming it. Meat rots in our system for maybe two or three days. Dogs, for example, have a short path to eat and discharge waste – their enzymes can dissolve bones. *Nature is telling us – are we listening?*

Humans and animals have skin to protect from outside elements. Even plant-based items don't want to be eaten! For example, onions have chemicals in their cells that throw out toxins when we cut them. Lentils and beans also have a coating that protects from "them being eaten"- called lectin. So, how to eliminate lectin – soak in water overnight and use a pressure cooker, such as an Instant Pot-type tool to cook under pressure. Such practical reasons and solutions are critical. Americans, in general, know little about the lentils – they know of only a half-dozen varieties! There are probably about three dozen lentils/combinations, which can be amazing possibilities for those on a plant-based diet.

Plant-Based Food: A Teaching Moment for the Public and Physicians.

Source: The Physicians Committee for responsible medicine, reported on 4 December 2020, *reported the following: (pcrm.org).*

"Albany, NY: New York State hospitals must make a healthful plant-based option available at every meal starting December 6, following a landmark bill that was signed into law last year. The Physicians' Committee for Responsible Medicine, which supported the bill, is a member of a nonprofit coalition that offers support, resources, and hands-on training to help hospital culinary teams provide more plant-based meals…this law gives physicians a teachable moment to discuss with patients the power of a plant-based meal to help prevent and reverse conditions like heart disease, diabetes, and obesity," says Susan Levin, M.S., R.D., director of nutrition education for the Physicians Committee. "Nearly 1.7 million New Yorkers have diabetes, and heart disease accounts for 40 percent of all deaths in New York State, according to the New York State Department of Health."

My Thoughts on Eating Certain Foods

My Single-Serve Sin

Mullah Nasruddin was born in present-day Turkey and died in the 13th century. He is considered a philosopher, Sufi, and wise man, remembered for his funny stories and anecdotes. He appears in thousands of stories, sometimes witty, sometimes wise, but often, too, a fool or the butt of a joke. A Nasruddin story usually has subtle humor. His stories are told in the entire Indian subcontinent and beyond.

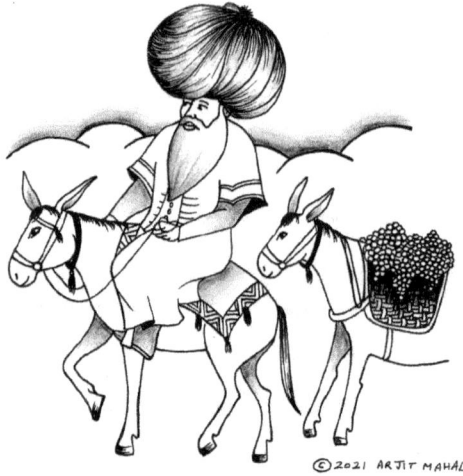

Figure 7.1 Mullah Nasruddin[13]

One of his stories goes thus: Mullah Nasruddin was going from one village to another to sell grapes. Grapes were loaded on his donkey. As he passed through another village, many children started to chase the donkey and asked the Mullah for some grapes to eat. The Mullah said to this crowd, "Do you remember last month when I passed this way, I gave you each some grapes to eat?" They all gestured in affirmative. Mullah asked them again,

---

[13] Source: https://en.wikipedia.org; Figure 7.2 Mullah Nasruddin is partially inspired by a 17th century miniature of Nasruddin, Topkapı Palace Museum Library.

"Do you remember the sweet taste of these grapes?" They all smiled and said, "Yes, they were heavenly." Mullah then said, "Well, these grapes taste the same, just close your eyes and sense that feeling of taste." With this advice, the Mullah moved on while the children were still sensing the taste with their eyes closed.

With my effort to reverse my diabetes, no matter how much I like something to eat, I use Mullah Nassrudin's approach. I don't deny myself anything, but I take just a little bit, a morsel of that delicious food, close my eyes and savor the taste from my memory. And say to myself, *I am full of this pleasure.*

I love ice cream. I take one spoon of it only, put it in my mouth, close my eyes, and savor it and say to my mind, *Hey, this was great, I just had a cup full of ice cream.* The mind settles down, and I win. I do the same with one potato chip, one cookie, one bite of pumpkin pie, one shot of Cognac or a glass of red wine, or anything else I have the desire for (remember it is a desire; not need!). I call it my single-serve-sin. (Remember, mind over matter!)

Eggs: The Scrambled Dilemma

There was once a teacher of law in old Athens. Students used to come to learn law from far and wide. The teacher had a policy of taking one-half of the fee upfront and the agreement would be made that the student would pay the second half when he would win his first case in a court of law. The school was successful. At one time, a student signed up for studies and paid one-half of the fee. After graduation, however, he decided not to practice law and did not pay the second half of the fee to the teacher.

The teacher, concerned about his fee, asked the graduate to come and see him. He told the graduate: "I am going to sue you in court. If I win, you will have to pay; and if you win and I lose, then per our original contract, you would have won your first case, and therefore you will have to pay anyway. So, why not just pay?" The law graduate replied: "Honorable Teacher, if you win your case against me, that means I would lose my first case in the court, and therefore, per our original agreement, I don't have to pay anything. If you lose the case against me, then it is clear, I won't have to pay at all, so why not just drop the case?" This is called a Dilemma!

With regards to eating eggs, I find myself in about the same situation as the law teacher and his student in old Athens.

I have a scrambled egg dilemma: To eat or not to eat eggs?

The contradictory and confusing "Egg Dilemma":

Dr. Neal Barnard, in his book, *Reversing Diabetes*, writes:

"There are just two problems with eggs: the yolk and the white. The yolk is where cholesterol lurks, with around 200 milligrams in a single egg. That's similar to an eight-ounce steak. The yolk also holds fat, about five grams per egg. The white has problems of its own since it is essentially pure animal protein. As you know by now, animal protein can present problems for your kidneys, and you are better off with plant protein...."

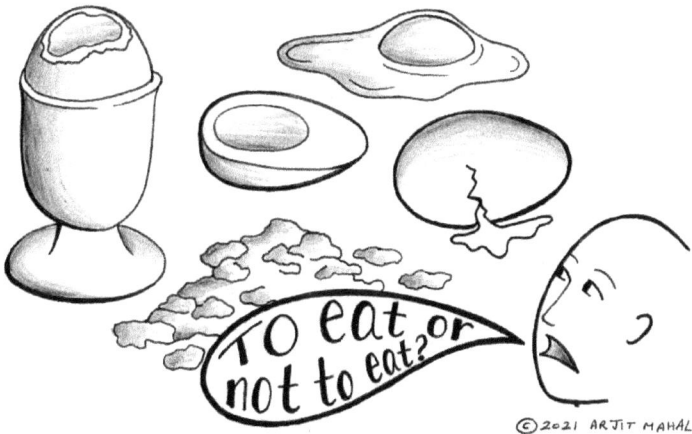

Figure 7.2 Scrambled Egg Dilemma

Dr. Dean Ornish's program on reversing heart disease allows egg whites (or substitutes), but not the yolk. His concern has been TMAO.

In *The New York Times*, the following article appeared on April 24, 2013. Here is an extract that gets into the "TMAO process." Eggs, Too, May Provoke Bacteria to Raise Heart Risk, By Gina Kolata.

"For the second time in a matter of weeks, a group of researchers reported a link between the food people eat and bacteria in the intestines that can increase the risk of heart attacks.

"Heart disease perhaps involves microbes in our gut," said the study's lead researcher, Dr. Stanley Hazen, chairman of the department of cellular and molecular medicine at the Cleveland Clinic Lerner Research Institute. In the case of eggs, the chain of events starts when the body digests lecithin, breaking it into its constituent parts, including the chemical choline. Intestinal bacteria metabolize choline and release a substance that the liver converts to a chemical known as TMAO for trimethylamine N-oxide. High levels of TMAO in the blood are linked to an increased risk of heart attack and stroke. To show the effect of eggs on TMAO, Dr. Hazen asked volunteers to eat two hard-boiled eggs. They ended up with more TMAO in their blood. But if they first took an antibiotic to wipe out intestinal bacteria, eggs did not have that effect.

Dr. Jason Fung, in his book, *The Obesity Code*, writes: "Eggs, previously shunned due to cholesterol concerns, can be enjoyed in a variety of ways: scrambled, over easy, sunny side up, hard-boiled, soft-boiled, or poached. Egg whites are high in protein, and the yolk contains many vitamins and minerals, including choline and selenium. Eggs are a particularly good source of lutein and zeaxanthin, antioxidants that may help protect against eye problems such as macular degeneration and cataracts. The cholesterol in eggs may actually help your cholesterol profile by changing cholesterol particles to larger, less atherogenic particles. Indeed, large epidemiologic studies have failed to link increased egg consumption to increased heart disease. Most of all, eat eggs because they are a delicious, whole, unprocessed food…egg yolks, once reviled as being high in cholesterol, have been vindicated. Studies now conclude that eggs, even daily, do not raise the risk of heart disease. In fact, consuming lots of eggs reduced the risk of diabetes by 42 percent." (references: Shin JY, et al. Egg consumption in relation to risk of CHD. Am J Clin Nutr. 2013 July 908(1): 146-159.)

In a *TIME* article on March 15, 2019, Jamie Ducharme reported the following: "Whether dietary cholesterol is associated with cardiovascular disease or death has been debated for decades. Positive, negative, and [neutral] associations have been reported," wrote study co-author Victor Wenze Zhong, a postdoctoral fellow in the department of preventive medicine at Northwestern University's Feinberg School of Medicine, in an email to *TIME*. "The existing literature is still controversial and inconclusive for nutrition experts and researchers to conclude the safety of eggs." She further goes on: "But yolks are the primary source of many nutrients found in eggs, including amino acids, iron and choline, so there is a downside to dropping them. Yolks are also one of the only natural sources of vitamin D, which many Americans lack...The research on eggs is contradictory—for now—so people (and their doctors) must personally decide how many eggs is too many, Zhong says. Those who are already at risk of cardiovascular issues may want to be more cautious than those who aren't, especially if they have a family or medical history of heart disease...."

Yet another study published on April 25, 2017, in the News Release in the Newsroom, a resource for journalists and medical outlets by Cleveland Clinic, states:

Cleveland Clinic Researchers First to Show Dietary Choline and Gut Bacteria By-product Linked with Increased Blood Clotting Risk, Heart Disease. A study published in AHA's journal Circulation also found aspirin may reduce the risk Cleveland Clinic researchers have shown, for the first time in humans, that choline – a nutrient typically found in egg yolks, red meat and processed meats, but dispensed via supplements in the study – is directly linked to increased production of a gut bacteria byproduct that increases the risk of blood-clotting events like heart attack and stroke. However, the research also showed that adding a low dose of aspirin may reduce that risk.

Enough on the Egg Dilemma!

If the reader is wondering why I have gone into so much detail on the egg issue, it is because I like eggs, and I have found that when I eat one egg, say in the morning, it helps keep my glucose numbers lower. In addition, it helps me sustain my fasting period. For now, I am taking a middle ground in that on alternate days, I may eat only the egg white and sometimes the full egg. (This is the reason also that I don't call myself vegan; vegans don't eat eggs).

I will keep a watch for the final word. One of these days, a scientist might unscramble this egg dilemma and get a Nobel Prize!

Apple Cider Vinegar

I am a fan of apple cider vinegar and use it effectively in a couple of different ways. I believe that it helps in my diabetes management in addition to general health. I can't prove this, but an inflamed blood vessel state caused by glucose may need the acidic treatment to cool it down.

Per WebMD:[14]

Apple cider vinegar is fermented juice from crushed apples. Like apple juice, apple cider vinegar may contain

---

[14]https://wb.md/2SErAs7.

various vitamins and minerals, as well as dietary fiber. Apple cider vinegar may also contain acetic acid and citric acid. It contains... nutrients such as B vitamins and vitamin C... Apple cider vinegar might help lower blood sugar levels in people with diabetes by changing how foods get absorbed from the gut. Apple cider vinegar might prevent the breakdown of some foods.

Typically, I buy unfiltered, unpasteurized, made from organic apples, with "The Mother." Most store-bought apple cider vinegar does not include the mother in the bottling process because it has been filtered and distilled out during the pasteurization process. However, if you buy raw vinegar, you will notice that there is a floating cloudy film at the bottom of the bottle. That substance is called the Mother. According to *The Journal of the American College of Nutrition*, raw vinegar contains probiotics, enzymes, and nutrients, which are good for health. My regimen is as follows: First thing in the morning, upon getting up, I drink two glasses of warm water to "wake up" my organs, so to speak. In one glass, I put some apple cider vinegar. I believe it is good for general health, but I have not done any extensive research in this area. It simply feels good. Prior to a meal (my main meal is mid-day), I drink apple cider vinegar with a glass of warm water before eating. I understand that it helps break down carbohydrates in food.

The most important benefit I have experienced is drinking diluted apple cider vinegar before going to bed. (one ounce or three tablespoons). I have found that when blood sugar rises in the morning, the spike is less than usual. For example, if by 8 a.m., I have had my blood reading say around 160, with the apple cider routine, the reading may be about 145, i.e., some 15 points, or say 10 percent less (learned from Dr. Fung's book). This is great for glucose management. The reader should check with their physician and, of course, experiment on their own to gauge the effectiveness.

Chyawanprash Jam with herbs and spices

Chyawanprash is a cooked mixture of sugar, honey, ghee, Indian gooseberry (amla) jam, sesame oil, berries, cinnamon, cardamom, and various herbs and spices. It is prepared as per the instructions suggested in Ayurvedic texts. Chyawanprash is widely sold and consumed in India as a dietary supplement. Chyawanprash tastes sweet and sour at the same time. Chyavana Rishi (Sanskrit: च्यवन, *Cyavana*) was a sage who was known for his rejuvenation through a special herbal paste known as chyawanprash. The recipe of chyawanprash is mentioned in manuscripts written for the Ayurvedic method of treatment, which he first prepared. Chyawanprash is usually consumed directly. It can also be consumed along with warm water. (source: Wikipedia). I enjoy a spoon full of this as a supplement in my Buddha Bowl.

Kala Namak (Himalayan Black Salt)

Per Preeta Sinha of onegreenplanet.org, "Kala Namak has a very distinctive smell. The sulfur compounds cause the salt to smell like hard-boiled or rotten eggs. Indian black salt has been used since ancient times and is said to have been identified by Maharishi Charak, the father of Ayurvedic medicine around 300 B.C.E. There are anecdotal claims from Ayurvedic healers that this type of black salt can be therapeutic. Of course, anyone should check with their physicians before using black salt for medical purposes."

I use Kala Namak often for adding flavor to soup or vegetable stocks that I may eat while fasting (It provides a certain satisfaction to the empty stomach). Many people find the pungent rotten egg smell to be offensive; it is an acquired taste. Most people from the Indian sub-continent are used to this salt as it is used in various types of cuisine and in Ayurvedic treatments and products.

Legumes & Lentils

In general, legumes are a class of vegetables that includes beans, peas, and lentils (aka Pulses or daals). The term lentil comes from the Latin word coined in the 1600s: "Lens.," named for the double convex glass (both sides curving outward). These foods are versatile in many ways for cooking, and their health benefits come with outstanding nutritional value. These are good for protein, fiber, and more and mostly have a low glycemic index. The legume family, among other benefits, is good for managing diabetes, heart health, and weight loss, plus fasting. I would refer to these as truly Mother-Earth-Jewels. For those who are vegans or prefer plant-based food, these should be the main item on their menus. My favorites are several lentils and beans such as chickpeas, with white and black and kidney beans.

Growing up on Punjabi food, *Daal* and *Roti* are embedded in my psyche. Daal is the name for lentils, and Roti is the Indian-style flatbread. Of course, there are other accompaniments such as *Sabzi* (cooked vegetables with spices), *Saag* (cooked mustard leaves), and *Makki Roti* (Corn Roti). My wife can tell you after being married to me for 50 years: "You can take a Punjabi out of Punjab, but you can't take *Daal-Roti*, out of a Punjabi." This is true for all cultures; the foods they grow up with would be part of their psyche.

Sheikh Saadi, Abū-Muhammad Muslih al-Dīn bin Abdallāh Shīrāzī better known as *Saadi of Shiraz*, was a well-known Persian poet and prose writer of the medieval period, in present-day Iran. He was admired for the depth of his social and moral thoughts. He used to be revered by people wherever he traveled, and they would throw banquets in his honor with the best possible foods they could muster. On his travels to the Indus Valley from across the Khyber Pass of Afghanistan, after eating his meals, he would always say, *"Wah Davte Shiraz!"* ("Oh, my banquet of Shiraz, this food is nothing like that.") The hosts were perplexed at what could be better than what they had served? On one occasion, a person visited Saadi's home in Shiraz and was curious to taste the great food Saadi had always mentioned. The visitor was invited in front of a kitchen fireplace in a simple room with simple furniture to sit down for meals. The servants served them *Daal and Roti.* Saadi said, *"This is Davte Shiraz,"* the best possible banquet.

The simple meals that you grow up with are closer to your heart, mind, and soul!

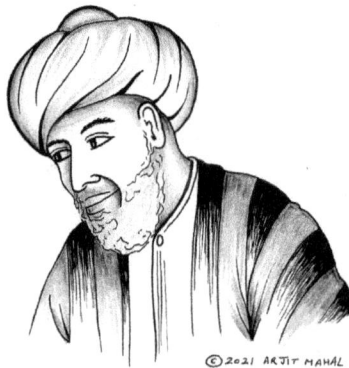

Figure 7.3 Sheikh Saadi

Lentils/Daals and beans come in a variety of sizes, some small, some larger. Some are called "split" or "washed;"

they have their seed coat removed, and the inner part of the lentil, known as the cotyledon, is eaten. I use these for cooking. Split lentils cook much faster than whole lentils.

There are unlimited possibilities of cooking: some as curries, others as dried or with a thicker texture. The spices, called *Masalas,* add many more possibilities for taste and texture. These are mostly eaten with wheat roti or rice. There are, of course, numerous ways of cooking. The daals are washed in water to clean and in some cases, depending on the type of daal, they are soaked for some duration to soften them. Mostly the daals are Sautéd with a mixture of oil, onions, garlic, ginger, tomatoes, chilies, and spices to form what is referred to as the "Tarka". There are two methods to blend the daal and the "tarka": first, while the daal is being cooked in water, the "tarka" is separately prepared and dropped into the cooked daal. The second is where "tarka" is made first in a pan, then the daal is added to it along with water to cook together. The legumes, such as chickpeas, have a similar process—more or less.

In American and possibly in the western country supermarkets, there are only a few varieties of daals on the shelves. For someone on a vegan or plant-based diet, my advice is to shop at a large Indian grocery store. There are many varieties of daals and beans available. Also, there are prepackaged masalas, a mixture of spices ready to be used for Tarka. These are unique for types of daals or beans—to get a certain flavor and taste. For example, Chana Daal (split chickpeas), masala is called "Daal Masala," for chickpeas cooking, the masala is called "Chana Masala." However, a generic one called "Garam Masala" (hot masala), a mixture of various spices, can be used for any cooking. The easy way to learn is to watch various people who share their recipes on YouTube. There are many people demonstrating how to cook. Please note that ready-cooked daals and beans are available everywhere. However, for someone like me, on the Ornish Lifestyle Medicine Program, the pre-packed ones may not be good. Use them sparingly—if one must. Sprouted daals are also available in the marketplace; they are high in protein and easy to cook to taste.

One word of caution: Lectins are a naturally occurring protein found in most plants. Some foods that contain higher amounts of lectins include beans, lentils, tomatoes, and potatoes. Lectins serve a protective function for plants as they grow. The same features that lectins use to defend plants in nature may cause problems during human digestion. They resist being broken down in the gut (they also don't want to be eaten…just as we humans don't want to be eaten by animals!). Lectins are water-soluble. They become inactive by soaking in water, boiling, or stewing. Now, I understood why our mothers and grandmothers in Punjab used to soak the daals and beans, sometimes overnight, depending on the type of daal. I also roast nuts such as walnuts and almonds for the same reason—to avoid lectins (in case they have it).

Sprouted Lentils: Sprouting Lentils are a powerhouse of protein and other nutrients: a living, fresh, and delicious source of enzymes, proteins, and minerals. Most of the nutritional advantages to the body are suppressed by anti-nutrients (phytic acid). Per Harvard School of Public Health's T. H. Chan: "sprouting neutralizes phytic acid and facilitates the bioavailability of nutrients like B vitamins and vitamin C, and more." When you sprout, the lentil comes to life and releases its innate energy which is easy for digestion and for the assimilation of nutrients.

I have found that sprouted daal is easy to cook (this when purchased already sprouted; sprouting can be done at home). For snacks and even for the main meal, first, soak the sprouted lentil in water for a couple of hours, then cook in boiling water until it is not hard but still crunchy. Then some simple spices can be added to taste. They give a feeling of fullness when eaten, and they do not spike post-meal blood sugar as much. While fasting, if I need a small snack to hold me, sprouted cooked daal is handy.

Fruits

Dr. Richard K. Bernstein, in his book, *Diabetes Solutions: A Complete Guide to Achieving Normal Blood Sugars. Little, Brwon And Copmany (2011).* gives the following advice, which has made sense to me, and I continue to follow his advice on eating fruit.

"...eliminating fruit and fruit juices from the diet can initially be a big sacrifice for many of my patients. They usually get used to this rapidly, and they appreciate the effect on blood sugar control. I haven't eaten fruit in over forty years, and I haven't suffered in any respect. Some people fear that they will lose important nutrients by eliminating fruit, but they shouldn't be worried. <u>Nutrients found in fruits are also present in the vegetables you can safely eat.</u>"

Dr Bernstein further provides advice on vegetables as a good alternative for diabetics: "...In our society, we generally reserve the name "fruit" for sweet fruits, such as apples, oranges, and bananas, all of which you should avoid. There are, however, a number of biological fruits (the part of certain plants that contains pulp and seeds) that are benign for the diabetic, such as summer squash, cucumbers (including many types of pickles), eggplant, bell and chili peppers, and avocados. These tend to have a large amount of cellulose, an indigestible fiber, rather than a fast-acting carbohydrate. (It's worth noting that cellulose, found in vegetables and fruits, is essentially the same fiber that makes up much of the shady elm on the corner. It has indigestible calories our bodies won't metabolize because we don't have the enzymes to break down the special cellulose chains of sugars into digestible form."

Author's Note: Diabetics may want to be aware that once cooked, some "vegetables" have a higher glycemic index when compared to the raw state, including items such as carrots, corn, potatoes, beet root, and even onions. For example, raw carrots have a GI (Glycemic Index) of 16, but when the carrots are peeled, boiled, etc., the GI could go from 33 to 60. A good source of checking GI is the University of Sydney Glycemic index Website: http://glycemicindex.com/index.php.

Buddha Bowl

As stated earlier, Buddha Bowl is a popular name used these days for a plant-based vegetarian food bowl filled with healthy and colorful complete meals including fresh vegetables, grains, proteins, and other nutritious items— per individual taste. The animal products are excluded from this bowl (see Figure 7.4 Buddha Bowl). It is likely that this term is based on the bowls which the Buddhist Bhikshu's carried from door-to-door for alms, per their belief in a simple life. Bhikshu, Bhiksu, (Sanskrit) /Bhikkhu (Pali), is a Buddhist disciple who has taken the life of monastic precepts; a man who has given up the Householder's Life to live a Life of heightened virtue, in accordance with Buddhist precepts.

In my new lifestyle of plant-based good nutritious food combined with my fasting effort, I enjoy calling my food bowl "My Buddha Bowl." I take time to fill it with small quantities of items I would like to eat. One of the main benefits of fasting is that I look forward to my main meal, which may have been after 18 hours or sometimes 24 hours.

The ritual of assembling my Buddha Bowl and eating with mindful presence is altogether a new experience for me. Each morsel in the mouth has a distinct taste and aroma, which I was never aware of all my life. Now, I wonder how I could have gone about all those years without the true pleasure of enjoying Mother-Earth's noble nourishment gifted to us by nature! Figure 7.5, My Buddha Bowl, is an example of one of my meals: It contains tomatoes, pickled cucumbers, pickled onions, pickled ginger, sauerkraut, radishes, mushrooms, a dried fig or date, and a bowl of cooked sprouted *Mung Daal*.

Mother Earth Diet

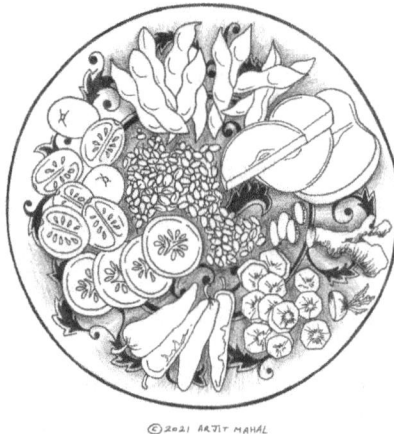

©2021 ARJIT MAHAL

Figure 7.4 Buddha Bowl

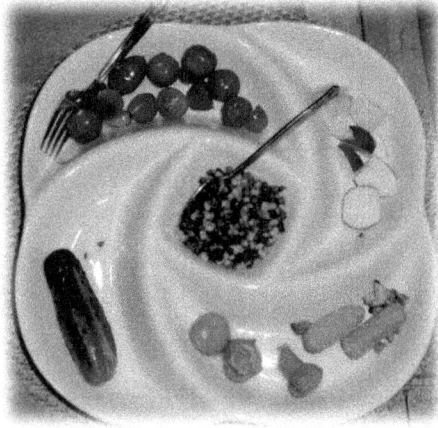

Figure 7.5 My Buddha Bowl

On Vitamins and Supplements

This is a complicated topic, and I would only mention that everyone's body may have unique needs based on his/her health, diet, or culture. Notwithstanding many articles that caution vegans and those on plant-based diets that there could be deficiencies in vitamins and minerals. I take the following supplements: Multivitamins, Cocoavia, Cocoa Extract Supplement, Alpha Lipoic Acid, Iron, Vitamin C, Vitamin D, Vitamin E, Vitamin B12, and Omega-3 (pure/prescription). On an ongoing basis, I assess the need for vitamins and supplements and adjust accordingly. As stated earlier, one must keep a balance stay within moderation (check with someone knowledgeable in this aspect).

This leads me to the next step in my transformation story.

Me, Cooking?

For half a century, my good wife has cooked for me. She learned Indian cooking; even though she was not born into that food culture, she became a good cook. The only thing I could cook was a fried egg or make a cup of tea. Sometimes when she would ask me to watch over and mix whatever she was cooking, I would hate that. She would always say, "You don't have patience...you should learn cooking; someday, you may have a need for it." She was right all along.

In the reversing heart disease program, a nutritionist would go into detail about plant-based food, the ingredients, the recipes, and methods of cooking without oils, introducing ingredients recommended in the Ornish Program. The executive chef used to make many recipes, and we, the cohorts, would eat together at lunchtime. They even introduced us to various practical utensils and demonstrated cooking techniques.

At home, I started to ask my wife not to use oils for cooking and declared that I would not have animal products: no cheese, milk, salad dressing with oils, or fish (I used to love fried shrimp). Since she was not in the

Ornish Program, it was challenging for me to defend why and what of this new regimen—every day of the nine-week course. One day, my subconscious told me to "take charge of your own food," and my mind said, "yes, you can do it!"

That is when I started to read about my favorite daals, their types, and cooking methods. My wife showed me how to chop onions and introduced me to basic cooking processes. My sisters and friends gave me additional orientation on some nuances of spices and the Tarka. (I still can't cut onions as small a size as my wife has been suggesting...I have a fear of ending up in the emergency room.) I cooked one daal (split chickpeas), and it came out very tasty. Then I tried making vegetable soup, and that was even better. Now I had control of what I wanted to eat, with what ingredients I wanted to use, and with what utensils I wanted to cook. My friend had introduced me to Instant Pot (sophisticated pressure cooker), but my wife still preferred to cook in a slow cooker. This disagreement was a blessing in disguise because she let me loose in the kitchen. One time she had commented on one of my daals: "it really came out good; the spices are just right, and the taste is the way it should be."

I had arrived in the kitchen!

This transformation helped me develop an appreciation for cooking including cutting vegetables, learning to prepare for and make a final product, such as daals, beans, masala-vegetables, and soups. I developed patience for this process and realized that it was therapeutic and meditative. Moreover, I learned that when you cook yourself, no matter what you cook, it tastes good and is always satisfying.

Depending on the cuisine, while many cultures around the world cook lentils and beans in a variety of ways, I am most familiar with what I cook now: daals and beans. The daal recipe in this book is more for my friends in the West who may be vegans, or on plant-based diets. This may expose them to wider options of basic Indian cuisine.

There are two sections under cooking: 1. Cooking Indian generic daal recipe—starting with learning about the basic step of making tarka/sauté; and 2. General recipes which I have learned to make from my family and friends. Some of these I have labeled after their names—to honor their contribution to my learning. These recipes are what I prefer to call experimental recipes. I don't go into the details of specific measures and precise details. A traditional style of recipe writing is out of scope for me. I suggest the reader get the idea and experiment. That is how I have learned. Good luck.

Tarka/Sauté

Before I start, the term and the concept of *Tarka* is important to understand in Indian cooking. This is typically the base of all daals, beans, and vegetables—cooked with spices. In her own words: An engineer turned food writer, Monica Bhide, writes about food and its effect on our lives. She is also the author of the book *Modern Spice: Inspired Indian Flavors for the Contemporary Kitchen* (Simon & Schuster). Following is her article, *The Crackling Spices of Indian Tempering*, on December 7, 2020, Guardian, narrated by Sala Kannan of NPR (National Public Radio).

"**Tarka**...Hot fat has an amazing ability to extract and retain the essence, aroma, and flavor of spices and herbs and then carry this essence with it when it is added to a dish. Tarka translates as "tempering." It is a method widely used in Indian cuisine, in which whole or ground spices are heated in hot oil or ghee, and the mixture is added to a dish. Hot fat has an amazing ability to extract and retain the essence, aroma, and flavor of spices and herbs and then carry this essence with it when it is added to a dish. American cooks are familiar with tempering as a way of heating and cooling chocolate. No relation. Indian tempering is done either at the beginning of the cooking process or as a final flavoring at the end. For example, when making a simple dish of rice with cumin, heat the whole cumin seeds in hot oil and then add the rice and continue cooking it. Tempering also can be used at the end of the cooking process. When making curd rice, for example, prepare the rice first and then, just before serving, temper it with seasoned ghee. I make this tarka by heating the ghee in a tiny skillet and seasoning it with crushed red chilies, garlic and mustard seeds..."

(Note: Those who are on a vegan and plant-based diet, substitute the ghee for something else, like olive oil spray and/or vegetable stock for making *Tarka aka Sauté).*

The following recipe is what I am going to refer to as the *Daal/Bean, Indian Cooking Recipe Template.* The reason is clear: there are so many permutations and combinations of ingredients and cooking methods—depending upon the geographic regions, that it cannot be covered in this book—nor do I claim expertise in that art. I am providing a basic recipe for North Indian Style Cooking. This template may be considered experimental. Try and improvise—as you like.

Daal or Bean Recipe Template

This recipe is a basic template. The time of cooking depends on the type of ingredients, spices, and taste, and preferred flavor and aroma. For this example, let us say we are going to cook Split Chickpeas Daal (it is yellow in color). The cooking time in a slow cooker will be more, a few hours, and in an Instant Pot, it may be just 30 minutes. To experiment, I started with a mixture of two daals: Mung (yellowish) and Masar (pink), both with the husk taken off. These are fast cooking daals and don't need a pressure cooker.

Preparation: Clean the daal from any debris (depends on where you buy it from), say one standard cup, in water, preferably three to five times until the water becomes somewhat clear. Soak the daal for about one to two hours in water. (Later, don't use the water it is soaked in.) If it is cooked in Instant Pot, soaking may not be necessary.

Get Spices Ready: Listed in the process (Indian names of spices are in brackets/parenthesis).

Wash/Cut Ingredients: Wash those needed to be washed and cut them into small pieces: onion, tomatoes, green chilies, ginger, and garlic.

Cooking Utensil: Preferred approach: wok or slow cooker or a pressure cooker e.g., Instant Pot

Process:

1. Put some olive oil in the preferred pan (or spray), on slow heat, and start the *Tarka*. (Those not using oil can use a spray can of olive oil or canola oil or substitute with vegetable stock.)

2. Put one teaspoon of Cumin Seeds (Jeera) in it and heat until it starts to get brown and emits an aroma—but do not burn.

3. Put onions in the pan and cook till they become brown. Here there are two approaches. If you put some salt in it, the onions will give out the water

quicker and get brown; but remember not to put salt later in the process. The other method is to hold off putting salt until later combined with all spices.

4. Add green chilies (two or three to taste) to the *Tarka*, followed by ginger and garlic. Ensure that these are well mixed /blended in the whole.

5. Add all spices: Measure according to taste. Preferably one-half teaspoon of each: garam masala (It is a mixture of some "hot" spices), turmeric (Haldi), red chili powder, salt, black pepper powder, coriander powder (Dhania). Mix well and let it simmer. Note: in some daals, such as the Black Daal (*Kali Mah di Daal*), it is advisable to put a pinch of Asafoetida (Heeng), which eliminates its gassy effect.

6. Add chopped tomatoes (tomato paste can be used as well) and let it simmer till the *Tarka* starts to "separate" and has been totally amalgamated (you start to see bubbles).

7. Add the soaked daal or beans. Add water, say for one cup of daal, add three to four cups of water. Let it cook for desired time (again, it depends on what tool is being used).

8. Check periodically to see the daal/beans are cooked enough. After that, keep on slow heat.

9. When done, add fresh coriander leaves (washed).

10. Ready to eat.

Basic Spices\Material for Indian Dishes

Aniseed (Saunf)	Cloves (laung)	Lentils (Daal)
Asafoetida (Heeng)	Coriander Leaves (Hara Dhania)	Mint (Pudina)
Bay Leaf (Tej Pattta)	Coriander Seeds (Sukha Dhania)	Mustard (Rai, Sarson)
Black Pepper (Kali Mirch)	Cumin Seed (Jeera)	Onion (Pyaz)
Black Salt (Kala Namak)	Dried Ginger (Saunth)	Salt (Namak)
Cardamom (Elachi)	Fenugreek (Methi)	Tamrand (Imli)
Chilies (Lal Mirch)	Ginger (Adarak)	Tumeric (Haldi)
Cinnamon (Dalchini)	Green Chili (Hari Mirch)	

Table 7.1 Indian Food Spices

General Experimental Recipes

When I had just developed interest in learning how to cook, particularly for my plant-based-diet need, a long-time friend Margie came to visit us. She brought a bowl full of appetizing mixed beans salad which is a regular item in her household. She said it was simple to make. This is the first item I had learned to make from her. Since then, it is a regular item in our household as well. Here it is.

Margie's Mixed Beans Salad

Ingredients		
3 or 4 cans of beans (15.5 oz/439g each). Select any of these: chickpeas, black beans, dark kidney beans, pinto beans, red kidney beans, black eye peas. Select different colored beans for variety	Yellow/Orange sweet peppers	Balsamic Vinegar
	2 tablespoons Dijon mustard	Cayenne pepper
	Optional: 1 tablespoon olive oil	Kosher salt
	Red onions chopped	Carrot (slivers)

- Put all beans in a strainer under cold water and drain
- Chop the carrots, cut sweet peppers, and cut onions in small pieces
- Put the beans and the above chopped ingredients in a bowl and mix well
- Add balsamic vinegar (to soak reasonably well...but not too much); Add mustard, cayenne pepper and salt to taste
- Mix well and enjoy
- Optional. Additional spices and herbs such as coriander for taste and flavor. To make it hot and spicy, add chopped green chilies.

Millie's Winter Vegetable Soup

Ingredients			
Cabbage	Carrots	Turnips	Onions
Celery	Green Beans	Tomatoes	Parsley
Vegetable tock	Tomato Paste	Salt	Pepper (hot pepper flakes)
Optional - Potatoes	Can of Chickpeas - drained	Mushrooms - sliced	Dill

- Wash and cut all vegetables into medium pieces and put them in a large pot
- Add all other ingredients in the put at one time
- Add salt and pepper to taste
- Add vegetable stock – 2 or 3 containers
- Put the pot on high heat till the ingredients boil
- Lower the heat and let it simmer till the ingredients are soft

Johnny's Naan Pizza

Ingredients			
1 Naan bread	Tomato Sauce (Marinara)	Mushrooms	Red onions – thinly sliced
Garlic – finely chopped	Basil	Oregano	Hot pepper flakes

- Brush a bit of olive oil on the naan
- Reduce the tomato sauce so that it is not too runny
- Cut mushrooms into small pieces
- On the naan, spread the tomato sauce, then add mushrooms, onions, garlic
- Sprinkle hot pepper flakes and oregano to taste
- Preheat oven to 400 degrees. Bake the naan until done to taste

Artie's Italian Pasta

Ingredients			
10 to 12 Fresh ripe tomatoes	8 to 10 garlic cloves cut very small	15 to 20 Basil leaves cut small	1 Pound of pasta, any kind penne or linguine (must be imported from Italy. DeCecco is best)
About 0.25 cup of virgin olive oil			

- Cook pasta for one minute less than it says on the box and drain
- In a wok or large pan, heat oil until it starts to smoke
- In rapid succession, toss in garlic, tomatoes, pasta, and basil and toss it for about 30 seconds
- Serve with grated Italian cheese* and red wine*
- .* I avoid cheese but put very little olive oil. Those who are not on plant-based diet may add these items if they like.

Jasvir's Cabbage and Rice

Ingredients			
10 Baby carrots quartered	4 Broccoli heads cut into 4 pieces each	1 Cabbage medium head sliced thin	Onions medium to large pieces (use one half first and save the remaining half for later frying)
3/4 Cup Basmati Rice, boiled in a medium pot till done (when done, rinse in cold water and drain)		$1/2^{nd}$ Cup of Green Peas – not cooked (frozen can be used for ease)	

- Put some olive oil in a pan and add onions
- Add 1 tablespoon of garlic and carrots till soft (don't burn onions)
- Add broccoli and sauté (light fry)
- Add cabbage last
- Put salt, garam masala (Indian mixed spices), 1 tablespoon of cumin seeds and some hot pepper (no turmeric)
- Add green peas
- Add remaining second half of onions and mix well
- Sprinkle some soy sauce

Arjit's Egg-Whites Masala Omelet

Ingredients			
4 to 5 egg whites	Olive Oil Spray	Red chopped onions	Scallions (green onions) cut small
2 Green Chilies – cut small (makes it spicy)	Salt	Cayenne Pepper – just a pinch	Coriander Powder – a pinch
Fresh Coriander			

- Mix egg whites well
- Add all ingredients at one time and mix again
- Spray some olive oil in a frying pan and heat on medium heat
- Pour all egg white liquid and mixed ingredients in the pan and cover the pan
- When it appears, the top side is cooked, flip over the entire omelet till done (keep it moist)
- Enjoy with toasted bread

Arjit's Barley & Mushroom Soup - Using Instant Pot

Ingredients			
1 Cup Barley (quick-cooking)	Mushrooms (small pieces)	Celery cut into small pieces	Red Onions cut into small pieces
Olive Oil	Ginger	Garlic	Tomatoes (cut into small pieces)
Green chilies (cut very small) (spicy)	Black Pepper	Turmeric	Garam Masala
Sea Salt	Fresh Coriander	Balsamic Vinegar	Red Wine

- Warning: Follow the Operations manual for how to perform the SEALING and VENTING. This is critical for safety.
- Spray some olive oil in the pot (or put very little) and add inions and one-half teaspoon of salt and press the Sauté button. (salt extracts water from onions quickly).
- When the onions are lightly brown, add ginger, garlic, tomatoes, turmeric, garam masala, black pepper, green chilies and let it sauté a little.
- Shut the Sauté button; Add little red wine and balsamic vinegar
- **SEAL the pot**
- Press the button for high-pressure level. Set for 5 to 7 minutes. When done, shut the pressure and wait till safe to open (**VENT** to release pressure).
- Add fresh coriander and enjoy.

Kuki's Sprouted Bean Snack

Ingredients		
1 Cup of Sprouted Black Chickpeas or Mung Beans (Available fresh or dried. Adjust boiling time accordingly.)	Cumin seeds	Cayenne pepper
	Sea Salt	(Optional – Chat Masala, or substitute for any desired seasoning)

- Wash and drain the beans
- In a pot, boil the sprouted beans until they are soft
- In a separate pot, spray some olive oil and put a tablespoon of cumin seeds—and sauté lightly till the seeds become light brown and start to give aroma
- Add salt or any seasoning of choice
- Add the beans to the pot and mix well
- Add any seasoning of choice

Arjit's Quick Chickpeas Snack

Ingredients			
1 Can of Chickpeas (aka Garbanzo) Beans	Cumin Seeds	Sea Salt	Cayenne Pepper

- Drain the can of the liquid and rinse with cold water and drain
- In a separate pot, spray some olive oil and put ½ tablespoon of cumin seeds—and sauté lightly till the seeds become light brown and start to give aroma
- Add salt or any seasoning of choice
- Add the beans to the pot and mix well
- Add any seasoning of choice

Now that I have learned the basics of cooking, I must discuss fasting next. This is nature's drama of yin and yang!

CHAPTER 8

Fasting

Some men have thousands of reasons why they cannot do what they want to, when all they need is one reason why they can.

Willis R. Whitney, American chemist

There are two parts to this chapter: The first is an easy-to-understand article by Dr. Jason Fung on the description of the science and methodology of autophagy, based on Noble Laureate Yoshinori Ohsumi's research. The in-depth methodology of this topic is described in-depth in Dr. Fung's books.

The second Part outlines my own experience with fasting. I have laid it out in the form of a timeline that goes over the step-by-step approach that I have been following with successful accomplishments of my goals, thus yielding a better health profile.

Before we begin, let us understand who Yoshinori Ohsumi is and what he did: discovery of mechanisms for autophagy.

Summary: This year's Nobel Laureate discovered and elucidated mechanisms underlying autophagy, a fundamental process for degrading and recycling cellular components.

The word autophagy originates from the Greek words auto, meaning "self," and phagein, meaning "to eat." Thus, autophagy denotes "self-eating." This concept emerged during the 1960s, when researchers first observed that the cell could destroy its own contents by enclosing it in membranes, forming sack-like vesicles that were transported to a recycling compartment, called the lysosome, for degradation. Difficulties in studying the phenomenon meant that little was known until, in a series of brilliant experiments in the early 1990s, Yoshinori Ohsumi used baker's yeast to identify genes essential for autophagy. He then went on to elucidate the underlying mechanisms for autophagy in yeast and showed that similar sophisticated machinery is used in our cells.

Ohsumi's discoveries led to a new paradigm in our understanding of how the cell recycles its content. His discoveries opened the path to understanding the fundamental importance of autophagy in many physiological processes, such as in the adaptation to starvation or response to infection. Mutations in autophagy genes can cause disease, and the autophagic process is involved in several conditions including cancer and neurological disease.

Yoshinori Ohsumi was born 1945 in Fukuoka, Japan. He received a Ph.D. from the University of Tokyo in 1974. After spending three years at Rockefeller University, New York, USA, he returned to the University of Tokyo, where he established his research group in 1988. Since 2009, he has been a professor at the Tokyo Institute of Technology.[15]

How to renew your body: Fasting and Autophagy

October 5, 2016, by MD in Intermittent fasting By Dr. Jason Fung

Source: Diet Doctor: *How to Renew Your Body: Fasting and Autophagy,* **www.dietdoctor.com**

In 2016, the Nobel Assembly at Karolinska Institute awarded the Nobel Prize in Physiology or Medicine to Yoshinori Ohsumi for his discoveries of mechanisms for autophagy.

Autophagy is essentially the body's mechanism of getting rid of all the broken down, old cell machinery (organelles, proteins, and cell membranes) when there's no longer enough energy to sustain it. It is a regulated, orderly process to degrade and recycle cellular components.

---

[15] Source: https://www.nobelprize.org/prizes/medicine/2016/press-release/. Nobel Prize® is the registered trademark of the Nobel Foundation.

There is a similar, better-known process called apoptosis, also known as programmed cell death. Cells, after a certain number of divisions, are programmed to die. While this may sound kind of macabre at first, realize that this process is essential in maintaining good health. For example, suppose you own a car. You love this car. You have great memories in it. You love to ride it.

Dr. Fung in his article gives a metaphorical example of an old beat-up car which we may get rid of and replace with a better functioning car. He states that the same thing happens in the body.

Cells become old and junky. It is better that they be programmed to die when their useful life is done. It sounds really cruel, but that's life. That's the process of apoptosis, where cells are predestined to die after a certain amount of time.

The same process also happens at a sub-cellular level. You don't necessarily need to replace the entire car. Sometimes, you just need to replace the battery, throw out the old one and get a new one. This also happens in the cells. Instead of killing off the entire cell (apoptosis), you only want to replace some cell parts. That is the process of autophagy, where sub-cellular organelles are destroyed, and new ones are rebuilt to replace them. Old cell membranes, organelles and other cellular debris can be removed. This is done by sending it to the lysosome, which is a specialized organelle containing enzymes to degrade proteins.

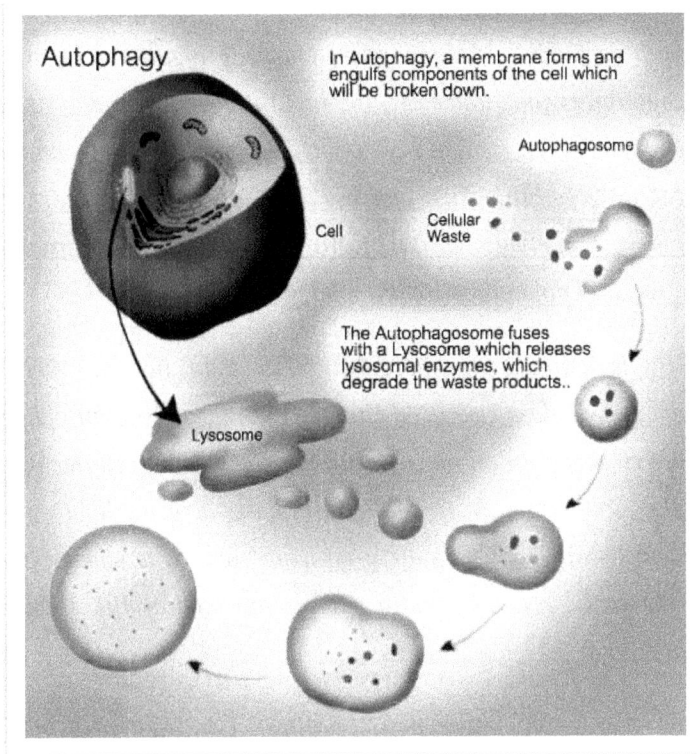

Figure 8.1 Autophagy Process

Autophagy was first described in 1962 when researchers noted an increase in the number of lysosomes (the part of the cell that destroys stuff) in rat liver cells after infusing glucagon. The Nobel Prize-winning scientist Christian de Duve coined the term autophagy. Damaged sub-cellular parts and unused proteins become marked for destruction and then sent to the lysosomes to finish the job.

Nutrient deprivation is the key activator of autophagy. Remember that glucagon is kind of the opposite hormone to insulin. It's like the game we played as kids – "opposite day." If insulin goes up, glucagon goes down. If insulin goes down, glucagon goes up. As we eat, the insulin goes up, and glucagon goes down. When we don't eat (fast), the insulin goes down, and glucagon goes up. This increase in glucagon stimulates the process of autophagy. In fact, fasting (raises glucagon) provides the greatest known boost to autophagy.

Fasting is actually far more beneficial than just stimulating autophagy. It does two good things. By stimulating autophagy, we are clearing out all our old, junky proteins and cellular parts. At the same time, fasting also stimulates a growth hormone, which tells our body to start producing some new snazzy parts for the body. We are really giving our bodies the complete renovation.

What turns off autophagy? Eating. Glucose, insulin (or decreased glucagon), and proteins all turn off this self-cleaning process. And it doesn't take much. Even a small amount of amino acid (leucine) could stop autophagy cold. So, this process of autophagy is unique to fasting – something not found in simple caloric restriction or dieting.

There is a balance here, of course. You get sick from too much autophagy as well as too little. This gets us back to the natural cycle of life – feast and fast. Not constant dieting. This allows for cell growth during eating and cellular cleansing during fasting – balance. Life is all about balance.

Inspired by Dr. Fung's and Yoshinori Ohsumi's research, the conceptual view in Figure 8.2 is the author's diagram to visually understand what goes on when we eat, when we stop and then start eating again. <u>When we eat, the insulin goes up, and glucagon goes down; when we don't eat, the insulin goes down, and the glucagon goes up. At this point, the self-cleaning process of autophagy is triggered into action</u>. The junky cellular parts are removed from the body, and the growth of new hormones stimulates the creation of body dells and parts. When we eat again, the autophagy shuts off.

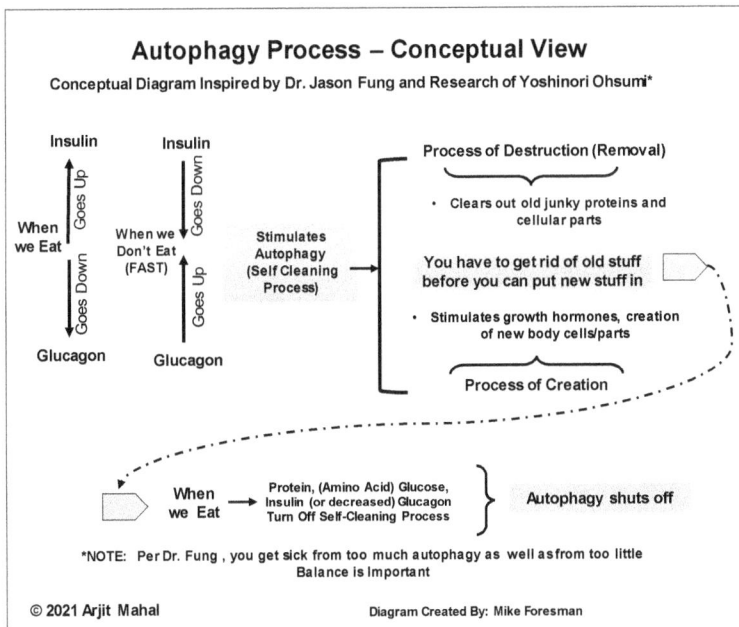

Figure 8.2 Autophagy Process – Conceptual View

My Experience with Fasting

There are books and articles on fasting referring to what is called "Intermittent Fasting" or "IF." Merriam-Webster Dictionary defines Intermittent as: "coming and going at intervals: not continuous; also: occasional." To me, the "intervals" can be an individual's choice of timeframes of eating and fasting—based on many factors, which include needing motivation, and such. This means that the intervals can be 12 hours, 18 hours, 24 hours, or a few days at a time. The fasting regimens are known by several titles, such as Whole-day fasting 5:2 which propose eating five days normally but restricting calories for next two days, Fasting 18-6 suggests fasting for 18 hours and eating only within the next six-hour window, Alternate-day fasting, Time-restricted feeding, or one-day-a-meal diet, branded by their originators as such.

Some authors who write about the 18-hour-fast state that after 18 hours, you should eat within the next six hours before you fast again; they also mention that in that six-hour eating period, you can eat whatever you desire, with no limit to the portion size of the food. While this may work for some people, for a person like me it would be a disaster to eat in that way. Why? Because if I as a diabetic did that, I would have to take extra medication or boost insulin intake to compensate for keeping sugar numbers in range. If one is trying to address their obesity problem or diabetes problem, the vicious cycle of increased food and insulin would invite more insulin resistance and weight gain, not to mention the effect on heart health.

I am not a fan of the term intermittent fasting because even normal meals eaten at intervals are intermittent, in my view. In the case of a person like myself who has three objectives: manage diabetes (undo it), heal heart (reverse disease contributing factors), and lower body weight, my approach for a fasting diet includes varying intervals with some food intake to "sustain fasting interval" and eating carefully planned foods when breaking the fast. If I were to name my approach, I would call Flexible Function-Fasting (FFF), but I will just label it "FF." (Maybe my name will go down in history with this brand!) The term "function" infers that the fasting diet is expected to perform some function for the body's homeostasis and thus well-being— irrespective of "intervals." Those are personal preferences based on one's own courage, commitment, and compliance. Terms make the difference in understanding the import of words.

After reading several books and articles on fasting, I started to get overwhelmed with all the details around their proposals. I put aside all that literature and decided that I would create my own fasting program by trial and error—for what would work for my temperament and body. I, however, found the following book to be very comprehensive and easy to understand for fasting: *The*

Complete Guide to Fasting, Heal Your Body Through Intermittent, Alternate-Day and Extended Fasting, by Jason Fung, MD, with Jimmy More.

My thinking was simple: I used to eat normally at 6 p.m. Then I would eat breakfast at say around 9 a.m. the next day. That would be 15 hours of fasting. So, that was already "Intermittent". Then I decided not to have breakfast till say 10 a.m. That meant I was fasting for 16 hours. Over the next few days, I pushed the time further to eating at 11 a.m. and then at noon. Now, I was fasting for 18 hours. Over the next few weeks, I realized that I really was not that hungry in the morning and could get by with a few walnuts, or a little protein-yogurt, or an egg, and have a meal at about 12:30 in the afternoon. The next meal would be dinner at 6 p.m.

I discovered that at my age, it was uncomfortable sleeping at night with the 6 p.m. so-called "main meal." Then I started to switch the food cycle. I made lunchtime, say about 12:30 in the afternoon, as my "main meal." At 6 p.m., I would have light soup, maybe some raw cut-up vegetables—and nothing else till the next day, 12:30 in the afternoon. So, I started to have my main meal at midday. Sometimes, at 6 p.m., I would simply have hot vegetable stock with a little kala namak (black salt) and red chili pepper for taste. As stated earlier, I sometimes switch the timing of my main meals, depending on the start and end of my fasting cycle.

With this pattern, my body started to get used to this approach, and I started to lose weight. In addition, I had more clarity in mind, I started to have more energy, and I would feel healthier in general. I did my best not to snack in between the two meals. However, I had to snack sometimes because the body "becomes stubborn" and "demands food," I would eat raw vegetables such as raw kohlrabi.

My sugar number stated to stabilize in my desired range. My need for insulin four times a day came down to only one time with a very low dose only. And if I exercised, even that low dose was not needed, provided I had a small portion of good-for-me food eaten so as not to run the risk of low sugar (hypoglycemia). This was, of course, all vegetarian food, with no animal products. This went on for a few weeks. My weight started to drop, and of course, the BMI started to come down.

My weight had come down from over 190 pounds to about 162 pounds. It stayed stuck at the number for weeks. I guess my body had reached its "set point." Then instead of what I call a 24-hour fast (with one main meal a day fast), I went on a 48-hour fast. To my amazement, my weight dropped by two pounds and came down to about 160 pounds. To me, it felt like breaking the "sound barrier" of set point. This was a new learning—and a happy one, giving me an "a-ha" moment!

My Experience with 24 and 48 Hours Fasting

As for the American families, Thanksgiving in November is an opportunity to express gratitude to the land of opportunity and its abundant gift to us for sustenance. It is a family affair. When I came to America as a student in 1968, living next door to my boarding house was a professor at Rutgers University. To introduce the meaning of and share in the spirit of this noble purpose, the professor invited a few of us students to his home for a Thanksgiving meal. Even though I did not like to eat meat, I tasted turkey for the first time and started to enjoy it annually on Thanksgiving Day.

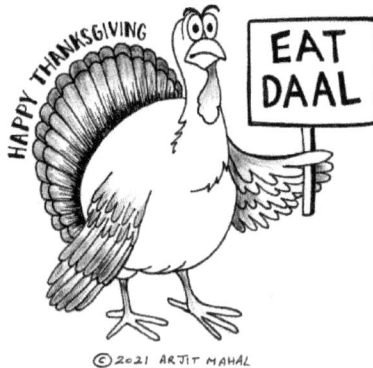

Figure 8.3 Thanksgiving Daal Slogan

Now 2020, since I don't eat any animal products, I still wanted to honor this special occasion to have a very small piece of turkey with gravy and wild rice—my typical favorites for that event. My wife had ordered a ready-to-eat Thanksgiving platter, from which I had taken a small piece of turkey. Fasting causes undue constraint on your spouse/partner during such a holiday when they want to enjoy their meals and don't want to be reminded of fasting and blood glucose issues.

After this traditional partaking of food, I decided to try a 48-hour fast. I outline below my diary of what happened, when, and how I felt, along with learning from the outcomes.

Precursor: I was on a 24-hour fast for a few days and had become confident that I could extend the time. The following experience is about 24 hours followed by another 24 hours, thus making a total of 48 plus fasting (I had extended it to a total of 53 hours).

24-Hour Fasting (First Day)

Time	Activity	Outcome/Learning
	Thanksgiving Holiday in the USA	
1:30 p DAY 1	Traditional lunch small piece of roasted turkey, gravy, sweet potato, wild rice, a forkful of pumpkin pie. A glass of water with some apple cider vinegar. Note: If it were not a holiday meal such as this one, I would have had my Buddha Bowl food: cooked or sprouted	I ensured it was not a heavy meal. Per Dr. Fung, apple cider vinegar helps to "cut" carbohydrates and helps balance blood glucose. While I have reduced my dependence on insulin, which I used to take four times a day, sometimes for a heavy meal, I

Time	Activity	Outcome/Learning
	lentils, with salad including pickled ginger, pickled cucumbers, radishes, and tomatoes.	take a small dose of insulin prior to the meal to ensure my glucose spike is manageable.
2:30 p	Conducted my daily routine of meditation, exercises, and rest.	This is based on the *Ornish Lifestyle Medicine* program with my own additional improvisations.
4:00 p	Black tea "Masala Chai"	I sometimes drink green tea. No milk or sugar was added.
5:00 p	Small drink: Cognac, total about four ounces. I have a habit of eating some salty snack with the drink.	This is my single-snack-sin: half a cup of snack mixture, often including roasted chickpeas and edamame.
6:00 p	Bowl of tomato soup	I was a bit hungry – but it was in the mind only.
8:00 p	Herbal tea with some salted almonds	Usually, I eat roasted walnuts and almonds as small snacks.

Time	Activity	Outcome/Learning
10:00 p	Preparation for sleep. Took water-diluted apple cider vinegar	Dr. Fung suggests in his book this technique of reducing blood spike in the early hours of the morning. In the early hours, the liver starts to put glucose in the blood to provide energy for the day's activities. In my case, at about 7 a.m., the glucose number would be about 160 and would keep on going up to 180 and beyond. Drinking diluted apple cider vinegar before bedtime reduced the numbers by about 15 points or about 10%. Sugar numbers started to be about 145 or so in the morning. The spike after that would be up to about 165/170. Dr. Fung is right: vinegar works.

Table 7.2 First 24 Hour Fasting Diary

My weight in the morning was 162.1 pounds, from the original of over 190 to 193 pounds at the beginning of 2019 (about 18 months ago). This was a remarkable achievement. While I was comfortable at this weight, I wanted to drop a few more pounds. However, for many weeks I was unable to drop the weight below 163 pounds. I assumed that it was my body's set point, and the body was resisting! I did not know how to overcome this issue.

The answer came to me when I went the next step to a continuous 48-hour fast.

Precursor: I had already been fasting for 24 hours. On the morning of the next day, my mind was telling me to eat a meal at midday. I did not feel hungry. I was full of energy and alertness. I had the courage to overcome my mind and decided to continue fasting for another 24 hours.

24-Hour Fasting (Second Day)

I have shown detailed blood sugar numbers for the benefit of those who may have diabetes. I want to be clear: I call my method of fasting Flexible Fasting (FF), because in a 24-hour period, while I have one main meal, I also take a little snack or vegetable broth when hungry a second time during this period. Listening to your body is important in fasting.

During the 52-hour fast, I had hunger pangs only twice, which I was able to handle with vegetable broth, or some nuts and one white only or whole egg. I felt "more alive" with energy, and there was no lethargy. I have been more energetic and mentally alert since I have started a regular fasting regimen. During this fasting, I had observed a particular smell in my urine and even in my mouth! I wonder if these were ketones or "cellular junk" exiting! (I have yet to find out, and this is the challenge. Who do you ask?)

Time	Activity	Outcome/Learning
Got up at 7:00a	Glucose Numbers: 3:00a: 100 5:30a: 130 11:30a: 157 and it stayed stable	When I get up in the night to go to the bathroom, I always check my blood glucose level. Thanks to my CGM monitor (more on this in Chapter 9. Tools) The other reason I check my blood at night is to ensure my numbers don't drop below, say 70 or so, risking hypoglycemia. Since eliminating long-term insulin intake before bed, I don't encounter this risk. However, it is a habit and not a bad idea to be alert. (I always have sugar tablets handy or Werther's Original Caramel Hard Candies to give some boost to sugar in the blood). But, because I had been on the new regimen of drinking two ounces of apple cider vinegar, I wanted to monitor my blood sugar closely.
2:30p	Started to feel some hunger. Had a bowl of vegetable stock. This portion was heated in the microwave, and eating slowly with mindfulness, dissipated my urge for hunger.	Dr. Fung suggests eating a bowl of bone stock with some salt. As a vegetarian, I prefer vegetable stock instead. It was satisfying. And the mind could not stray me to eat something else.

Time	Activity	Outcome/Learning
3:30p	Had Hot Green Tea.	No snack.
5:00p	Small drink: Cognac, total about four ounces.	Blood glucose number was 130. And I noticed that it did not significantly increase with one drink. (Sometimes, when in the mood, I may have a second drink, or instead, a glass or two of red wine—but no more).
6:00 pm	Glucose Numbers: 129	Glucose within a good range
7:00p	Feeling of hunger. Had a bowl of vegetable stock.	Observed: That vegetable stock does not increase blood glucose significantly.
8:00p	Herbal tea with some almonds and walnuts. Apple Juice two ounces	I don't drink juices as a norm; in some rare instances, I feel like having some, so I just drink a little bit (with constraint on the quantity; sometimes giving in to the mind is ok, humor it!)
10:00p	Preparation for sleep. Took water-diluted apple cider vinegar (small glass of about six ounces)	11:00p Went to bed

Time	Activity	Outcome/Learning
28 Nov	Glucose Numbers: 1:00a: 92 2:00a: 84 5:00a: 98 7:00a: 111 8:00a: 140	At 2:00a.m., I was concerned that while asleep, my blood count may not drop below 84. So, I took one glucose tablet. These over-the-counter tablets are good to keep handy for diabetics: 1 Tablet has only 4g of sugar (total of 4g carbohydrate). 1 Tablet raises glucose count by about 10. Alternatively, I keep Werther's Original Caramel Hard Candies handy. 1 Candy/Serving has about 4g sugar (total of 4g carbohydrate). I am currently exploring such single-serve candies made of pure maple syrup because the glycemic index of maple syrup is lower. Note: I carry such items on my person when I go out and have them in the glove compartment of my car. When fasting or otherwise, diabetics occasionally need such items to boost energy/sugar.
8:00a	Had two glasses of warm water with some apple cider vinegar in it	For years I have followed this practice to "wake up and cleanse the organs." (Ancient Ayurveda recommendation has been to use lemon juice).

Time	Activity	Outcome/Learning
9:00a	Started to feel hungry. Had about four walnuts and one boiled egg (whole with the yolk as well)	As discussed elsewhere in the book, the experts claim that egg yolk is not good for heart health, yet others claim that yolk is good for diabetics. A person such as myself who has both chronic conditions, Diabetes and Atherosclerosis, I guess, I must choose what body system to heal and preserve. For now, I have taken the middle ground. I eat an egg with yolk on alternate days. (maybe I can keep both body systems at peace...some humor is good for the mind!)
1:30p	Had a bowl of vegetable stock with salt in it.	At this time, I had been fasting for a total of 48 hours. I was not hungry and had no hunger pangs. So, I decided why not push fasting till 6p and join my wife for dinner. (One must accommodate the needs of family members as well, rather than isolate oneself). I was able to do this.
6:00p	Broke 52 hours of Fast with a decent meal of my liking	I felt a sense of accomplishment and proved to myself that it is not hard to fast for 48 hours. In fact, I could have continued for another day. Thus, I started to think that I need to schedule a 24-hour fast periodically and maybe do a 48-hour fast on occasion.

Time	Activity	Outcome/Learning
6:00 a Next Day	Bravo! My weight was 159.9	After weeks of not being able to go below 162 to 163 pounds, my weight for the first came down to 159.9 Lbs. This was equivalent to "Breaking the Sound Barrier" for me or breaking the "weight barrier." Could it be that I have been able to shift the body set point?

Table 7.3 Next 24 Hour Fasting Diary

During this fasting, the only negative feeling was a) I felt a bit "edgy" or "irritated" just before feeling hunger pangs; and b) Immediately after taking the vegetable broth, I had to go to the toilet. I don't understand the cause of this reaction. In any case, these issues are not show-stoppers for me. I am on for the marathon! I have also tried a 72-hours fast; after 48 hours of fast, the body and mind do not "pressure" you for food. I have not tried beyond this time frame. (Note: Sometimes, if I feel hunger pangs, I ignore it, and it goes away. This is proof for me that the mind wants its own way! But mind over matter works – with practice.)

Before and After Pictures – A Success

Pythagoras, Ancient Greek philosopher, mathematician had observed: "God built the universe on Numbers; Numbers rule the universe."

2019 & Before July 2020   2020 October & After

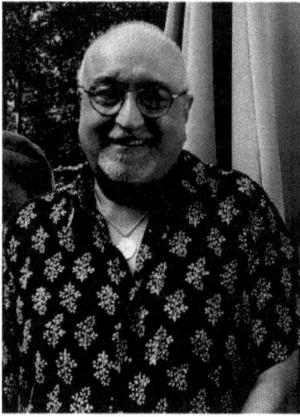

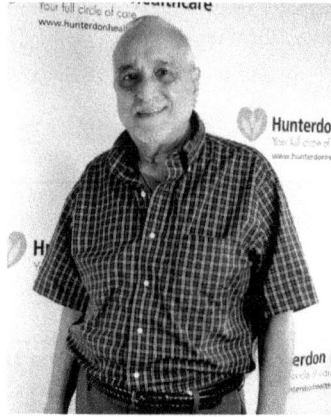

Figure 8.4 Arjit Before   Figure 8.5 Arjit After

Let us see what my before and after numbers show.

Here are my numbers of some key health indicators from my blood report. While I had started fasting at the beginning of 2020, this dramatic change shown below occurred after I had participated in the 9-Week Ornish Lifestyle Medicine Reversing Heart Disease Program. Prior to July 2020, while I had started the plant-based diet, I was still eating fish and using cooking oils in foods, so was not as disciplined—as I became later—thanks to the Ornish Program awareness and tools.

Comparison of Bloodwork Reports: July 2020 and October 2020.

Legend: ++ Measures are in mg/dL

Measures	July 2020	++	Oct. 2020	++	Reference Ranges are sourced from Quest Diagnostics' MyQuest Blood Work Report
Lipid Panel, Standard					
Cholesterol, Total	157	mg/dL	98	mg/dL	Reference Range: <200 mg/dL
HDL Cholesterol	38	Mg/dl	34	mg/dL *	Reference Range: > or = 40 mg/dL *This low number has genetically low. I am told this is genetic! The ration below "matters more!"
Cholesterol /HDL Ratio	4.1		2.9		Reference Range: <5.0 (calc)
LDL Cholesterol	90	Mg/dl	42	mg/dL	Reference Range: <100 mg/dL This indicator shows that Arteriosclerosis is "not progressing" (CHD) is in a better place.
Triglycerides	203	mg/dL	136	mg/dL	Reference Range: <150 mg/dL
Non-HDL Cholesterol	119	mg/dL	64	mg/dL	Reference Range: <130 mg/dL (calc)

Measures	July 2020	++	Oct. 2020	++	Reference Ranges are sourced from Quest Diagnostics' MyQuest Blood Work Report
HS-CRP	not tested		0.6 mg/L		Reference Range: Optimal <1.0 mg/dL Shows Inflammation is "in check".
Hemoglobin A1C	6.7%		7.1%*		Reference Range: <5.7 % of total Hgb *6.7 was with taking insulin four times a day; 7.1 is without taking any diabetic medication. For a Person my age, 7 to 8% is acceptable.
C-Peptide	1.42	ng/mL	2.03	ng/mL	Shows more insulin is being produced by the pancreas
Insulin Autoantibody	Not tested		13.1		Reference Range: <0.4 U/mL.
Weight in Pounds	190		170		Lost 30 pounds. (In Dec 2020, weight came down to 160 Lbs.)
BMI	28.5		25.5		A drop of 3 points. (In Dec 2020, BMI was 24.0)

Table 7.4 Blood Work Comparison

What I have learned by Fasting

Some days the body just demands food intake. Do it in a controlled way to avoid spiking the blood sugar. For example, I may eat a boiled egg with the yolk or sometimes without yolk. I have noticed that if my blood sugar was around 135 at 8 a.m. and if I ate an egg, the number may go up to 175 and stabilize. If I don't eat anything, the number may go up to 190 and even 200 before coming down. That means that a boiled egg with yolk has something in it that does not let the sugar spike as much, and it gives the satisfaction of fullness. Since I am hoping to cut eggs out of my diet, I am experimenting with alternatives for breakfast, such as oats.

Diabetes: My glucose numbers had significantly dropped. I had stopped taking insulin four times a day (a total of about 80 IUs, a combination of short and long-acting insulin regimens). Somedays, I had to take a small dose to manage my post-meal glucose spike. However, for my main meal, on rare occasions, I needed a small dose of medication.

The Heart: I have been mainly concerned with Atherosclerosis. If there is diabetes, there can be heart issues—these, along with hypertension, are "partners-in-crime," i.e., sometimes they go together. I had heart bypass surgery 24 years ago and had to have stents implanted. Over the years my blood profile had issues. I needed to bring the numbers to a reasonably safe number. I have achieved that successfully.

Weight: While I did not classify in the obese category, I was in the overweight category most of my adult life. Learning from various sources, it was the common medical sense that if I reduce weight, both diabetes and heart issues will be better managed. This was accomplished. (Note: now with my BMI at 24.0. I am in the normal category.)

General Well-being: My health objective has been to have and maintain quality of life in whatever time I may have on this earth. Simply put, quality of life over quantity of years. I am more energetic, more mentally alert; my dentist and dental hygienist of over 35 years state that my gums are "pink" and healthier; my skin seems to be healthier. Overall, I am pleased with my current health profile.

General Benefits of Fasting - I have experienced

- More energy (less lethargy); Body has more agility
- More mental clarity and concentration
- Lowered blood sugar levels
- LDL Level dropped (Bloodwork shows)
- LDL/HDL ration improved (Bloodwork shows)
- C-Reactive Protein – In range (marker of inflammation)
- Improved fat burning (weight loss is the proof)

- Reduced diabetes and blood pressure medications (blood glucose must be monitored diligently)

Some Challenges

"Hunger is a state of mind, not a state of stomach." Dr. Fung.

Continuously adjusting diet every day. It is manageable.

Participating in family meals and going to restaurants (have to plan ahead).

(Little humor: My clothes became baggy, so I gave away my old wardrobe. This is a good thing.)

Food & Cooking: My wife has been cooking for me for over 49 years, and I am grateful for that, and now I understand what it takes to run the kitchen since I have started to cook some basic items myself. I can plan and choose my needs: what I want, how I want, and when I want. Now I admire the effort that goes in for people who are solely managing cooking for their families. When you cook for your own self, no matter how it comes out—it always tastes good!

Free: Autophagy fasting is free. It does not cost anything; in fact, one saves money by eating less. One does not need a doctor's prescription or approval from any health insurance. One does not have to change wardrobe because of no weight gain. (however, one must discard those baggy clothes for better fitting clothes. So, this is a wash...zero-sum outcome.) In fasting, one is the master of one's own destiny! One can stop and go at will.

Eating Plan: With practice and time, your mind prompts you less to eat food at a whim. But it does create a pleasing anticipation to enjoy the meal to come after fasting. Every morning I plan what I am going to eat during the day. And, I mark on my calendar the days I would have a 24-hour fast or 48-hour fast or more. This helps my wife and I to plan our menus—which may be different based on our preferences; it helps our grocery purchase list; and, most importantly, the calendar is planned around family events or meals out. This way the spouse/partner and family members don't feel that they and I are not connected by a common purpose of enjoying meals together. This especially helps on special occasions such as birthdays, anniversaries, and such.

My Fasting Challenges

- **Fear** of what would happen and how would I not be able to eat for an extended time? (The lows encountered come in waves. They are manageable with experience and practice.)

- **Schedule.** Will I be able to skip breakfast and not eat in the time frames I have been accustomed to? (If usually, one does not feel hungry in the

morning, mostly it is in the "mind", maybe
psychological.)

- **Understanding.** Trying to make sense of all the
  fasting gurus' books. There are contradictions. Who
  to believe? This is where the Occam's Razor
  principles helped me narrow down the ideas to a
  reasonable, common-sense approach.

- **Lonely Journey.** Getting my spouse/partner on
  board with my new plant-based diet mission
  (Mother-Earth-Diet). She is a noble wife and soul
  and a friend of 49 years; and has taken care of me
  all these years in my ups and downs of diabetes
  and heart health issues. As she does not have
  health issues such as mine, I have a guilty feeling
  sometimes when I don't join her for meals.
  Sometimes, I had observed a sense of frustration in
  her voice when she would talk about what to cook
  as my habits in terms of nutrition, preparations,
  and portions had changed. Occasionally, even in
  food shopping, I sensed she was frustrated because
  of the change in meal plans. Some of our groceries
  come from bulk grocery stores. My wife asked me
  once: "if I buy the shrimp salad, will you share that
  meal with me?" "No," I replied. "Ohhh," she said
  and did not buy that item. While my wife has seen
  my achievement that shows in my weight loss and
  bloodwork results, I felt that she is put in a position

where she is compromising her pleasures of eating and enjoying. To manage her expectations, one day, it dawned on me that I should write a manifesto for her and have a "sit down." This worked well; my wife's attitude thereafter toward what I was trying to accomplish had become one of understanding and support. (See my Autophagy Manifesto at the end of this chapter.)

- **Cooking.** Learning about Mother Earth Foods to prepare for myself. I mostly eat Indian food, but I have not been familiar with the types of food items such as vegetables, lentils/beans, spices, oils, utensils, and recipes. (My wife coached me along with sisters and friends, and of course, "YouTube Cooks" are a good resource.)

Where Next – My Current Thoughts?

- **Future is unknown:** *You do not know what you don't know*! I may continue to have the quality of life that I am enjoying now, or there may be something around the bend that may cause concerns. My motto in this regard is the British WW2 slogan: *Keep Calm and Carry On.*

- **Barriers.** As I am a type 1.5 Diabetic (LADA), I know through testing that my insulin autoantibody is killing the insulin produced by my own pancreas. Interestingly, the injected insulin is not impacted by antibodies. Physicians tell me that antibodies are what they are, and any medication would cause complications with my autoimmune system. One of my physicians who has studied antibodies may get my blood tested for the type of *Antibody Arrays* I may have and then possibly figure out some solution. If that can be successful, then I can say that I have reversed diabetes 100%.

Once, the prime minister of Great Britain, Benjamin Disraeli, had this to say. Disraeli was physically challenged and had to walk with the help of crutches. One time, he asked his aid to do some task; to that the aid replied: "Sir, but that is impossible." "Impossible you say," Disraeli annoyed, pointing to his crutches, he said, "I walk on impossibilities every day."

- **Conviction**. Continue to have Courage, Commitment, and Compliance. "Damn the torpedoes; full speed ahead," as the WW2 American General said.

Hints & Tips

- **Coercion**. If your spouse/partner coincidentally can be in this program, that would be ideal. But forcing or trying to influence may not work.

- **Fasting does not mean eating nothing at all**. There are options: water, coffee, tea, vegetable broth, raw vegetables, and some nuts on occasion.

- **Don't tell anyone.** If you are fasting, keep it to yourself. Stephen R. Covey, educator, writer, and speaker, said it wisely: Most people do not listen with the intent to understand; they listen with the intent to reply.

- **Don't indulge** in conversations such as "let me tell you what is good for you!"

- **Don't try to explain** what various health gurus say about nutrition and autophagy regimen. You get challenged every step of the way. I have spent hundreds of hours understanding my health issues and healing possibilities by reading books and through other resources. I find myself rationally explaining the process, and the context, which the other party may not have any interest in (people are looking for "a quick answer"). I trust my own understanding and instinct. Those who are interested seriously, just refer them to resources— and let them invest their own time and energy in discovery. Besides, some people may have only one health issue, such as pre-diabetes, so, if I try to tell them the overall context, they do not want to hear the details. You can't tell people anything, especially when it can be controversial. The adage was, in other people's company, don't discuss religion and politics. Well, add Mother-Earth-food and fasting to that list.

(Note: You don't have to explain if you don't feel like it. It's okay to say, "I'm uncomfortable with your comment," and move on to something else. You're not required to explain if you'd rather be private.)

- **How much to share with your physician**? Notwithstanding sharing my health issues and medications openly with my health care providers, I don't try to tell too much if they show no interest in what I am doing to improve my health in terms of autophagy and fasting. I just discuss the results and outcomes. Unless, of course, he/she understands the concepts of Mother Earth foods and fasting and would ask questions, either because of motivation or for advancing their own professional self-development.

- **Monitor overall health and medications**. With weight loss, as the body's physiology changes, there can be consequences such as a drop in blood pressure. Then the medication has to be reduced as one example. My symptom was feeling light-headed upon getting up from a chair. Regular monitoring and tracking of my blood pressure numbers showed that I did not need the medication for this condition.

- **Mind Over Matter.** Always observe and prevent your mind from making mischief. It looks for an opportunity to make you stray from your activities and objectives. If you don't let it do what it wants, it backs off and leaves you alone for some time. But it is a continuous moment-to-moment event--watch over it.

- **Stay Engaged.** Stay busy with some activity you like. I am an author and have a few published books. Currently, I am writing a book on the history of an area of my interest. In between writing and writing blocks, rather than thinking of eating something, I started to write this very book. So, two books in parallel keep me well engaged in creativity. (Some humor: In writing, I can tell stories that I like—many these days don't have the desire to listen—they would rather reach out for their mobile devices.)

- **Quality of Effort:** A story goes, a disciple one day asked his Zen Master if he would meditate for eight hours in a day, how long it would take him to "transcend," i.e., attain Nirvana. Ten years was the master's response. The disciple asked again, what if he was to meditate 16 hours in a day, then how long will it take to "transcend"? Twenty years, the Master replied. The discipline was confused as to why it would take twice the time for meditating more hours. The Master stated that the purpose of life is to enjoy and find meaning; if one were to just put more hours, then one would have missed the point in what the purpose of life is. The message: It is not "quantity" but rather focus on "quality" matters. Similarly, in fasting, it is the quality of the process of fasting, not just counting hours.

- **Fit fasting into your own schedule** (that is why I like my term Flexible Fasting). Plan, when there are family meals or dinner out, is planned. While occasionally I may pick a small quantity of food that suits me, when visiting family or friends, I carry my own food. (some humor: If they start giving some argument that fasting or vegetarian foods may not be good, I ask them, "Do you know how long meat stays in your body after eating?" Questions stop immediately.)

- **On Fasting Days:** I drink coffee, lots of water with apple cider vinegar, vegetable stock with Kala Namak and some red pepper flakes. (It is satisfying).

- **Breakfast:** I discovered by practice that breakfast was not essential. I could fast from after dinner, say at 6 pm to the next day at noon—18 hours of fasting. In the early hours of the morning, our bodies invoke a process called the dawn phenomenon. It is part of the natural circadian rhythms, predictable physical, mental, and behavioral changes that follow a 24-hour cycle that tells the body when to sleep, wake, and eat. It provides enough energy to carry on till lunchtime.

- **Ghrelin, the hunger hormone,** according to Dr. Fung, rises and falls in a natural circadian rhythm. During an extended fast, the ghrelin peaks during the first two days and steadily falls after. I have experienced this feeling.

My Autophagy Manifesto

Dear Wife,

I have heart health issues for the last 25 years and diabetes for the past 15 years.

Surgeries and medications have helped me maintain my life as best as possible so I thought it was possible then!

After almost two years of self-study and research about my health issues, I have discovered some natural approaches to healing myself. As you know, I have embarked on this journey with possibility, hope and courage. My blood profile and weight reduction are proof that I am on the right track for my wellbeing.

While I can manage my challenge with courage, commitment, and compliance, I know that sometimes you find it frustrating because I cannot eat with you the type of foods we used to eat, where we used to eat and when we used to eat. The volumes of information on this topic I have studied are hard to explain in small snippets. If you ask me anything about my approach, I will explain my reasoning as best as I can without being technical (which I have limitations regarding medical know-how.)

I want you to know that you are my partner in this journey in many ways. You have always shown your concern for my health and wellbeing; you are coaching me in learning how to cook, and you are supportive of my efforts-always.

However, my new protocols of eating and sleeping may seem "odd", but I must do what I must do. One must try and fail rather than not try at all. **For me, failure is not an option.** I am going to "reverse" diabetes and heal my heart as much as possible.

There are times I will feel tense, moody, and edgy. This is not because I am angry at you or about any situation. It is because, in Fasting, the hunger comes in waves; they come and go in with the rhythms of the body's natural cycle. Part of it is the mind playing games with my effort, and I have to "harness" it moment by moment.

I sincerely thank you for your support, love and help in so many ways. If I succeed in my mission, you would have enabled my achievement. I express my gratitude for that.

Love

Arjit

CHAPTER 9

Tools

You are your best tool.

Arjit Mahal

To achieve bigger goals, one must identify smaller steps and make progress diligently to achieve the final vision. First, one must have the vision and establish or acquire tools to measure success. Second, stick to one's program. The data collected thus is helpful in one's understanding of the body, but it becomes an especially useful tool for the medical practitioners to get snapshots over time for diagnosis and treatment.

In this chapter, I share only the tools I use, not what is in the marketplace. The medications and supplements are out of scope, as those are adjusted for an individual's need.

My GOAL: "Reverse" Diabetes/Improve Insulin Sensitivity; Reverse Heart Disease Contributors; Lose Weight; Improve Health and Well-being

To achieve this goal, I have my own set of tools which are conceptually depicted in Figure 9.1 You Are Your Own Best Tool. The toolset is, of course, dependent on individual needs. However, the best tool is one's own self: the attitude, research, compliance, and a desire to better manage health and well-being.

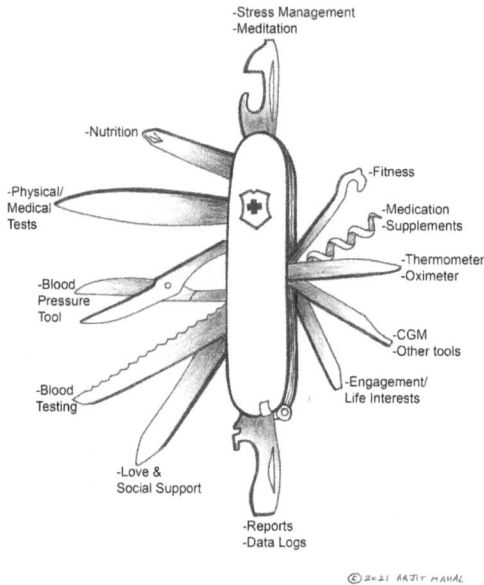

-Stress Management
-Meditation

-Nutrition

-Fitness

-Physical/
Medical
Tests

-Medication
-Supplements

-Thermometer
-Oximeter

-Blood
Pressure
Tool

-CGM
-Other tools

-Blood
Testing

-Engagement/
Life Interests

-Love &
Social Support

-Reports
-Data Logs

© 2021 ARJIT MAHAL

Figure 9.1 You Are Your Own Best Tool

Vitals

For trying to reverse diabetes, heal my heart, and lose weight, I have these devices that I use periodically and record the data.

Thermometer: I use a Non-contact Forehead Infrared Thermometer. Since it does not touch the body, it is more hygienic.

Oximeter: Pulse oximetry is a device put on the fingertip that measures the amount of oxygen in blood. It shows whether the heart and lungs supply enough to meet the body's needs. The pulse oximeter uses a special type of light to see how much oxygen is in the red blood cells traveling through the blood vessels under the skin. (*Source: WebMD*). This device also shows the pulse reading.

Blood Pressure: I use an Automatic Blood Pressure Monitor. It goes on the upper arm and is easy to use. There are other types available such as the one that goes on the wrist. The American Heart Association considers blood pressure normal when the top number is less than 120 (when the heart is contracting), and the bottom number is less than 80 (when the heart is relaxed).

Blood Pressure Categories

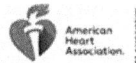

American Heart Association.

BLOOD PRESSURE CATEGORY	SYSTOLIC mm Hg (upper number)		DIASTOLIC mm Hg (lower number)
NORMAL	LESS THAN 120	and	LESS THAN 80
ELEVATED	120-129	and	LESS THAN 80
HIGH BLOOD PRESSURE (HYPERTENSION) STAGE 1	130-139	or	80-89
HIGH BLOOD PRESSURE (HYPERTENSION) STAGE 2	140 OR HIGHER	or	90 OR HIGHER
HYPERTENSIVE CRISIS (consult your doctor immediately)	HIGHER THAN 180	and/or	HIGHER THAN 120

heart.org/bplevels

Figure 9.2 Blood Pressure Measures

Note: Latest research shows that the blood pressure should be taken on both arms. The disparity in numbers may be indicators of potential health concerns. Physicians may be able to address this new thinking.

Glucose Monitoring

Just as in blood pressure, the following target blood sugar levels for the diabetes chart are important for self-awareness and diabetes management.

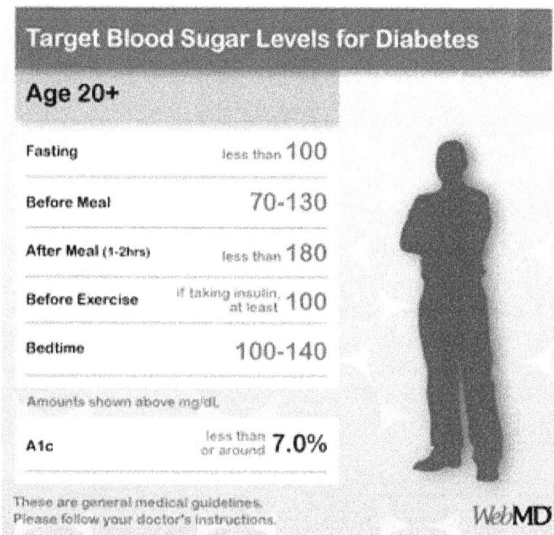

Target Blood Sugar Levels for Diabetes

Age 20+

Fasting	less than 100
Before Meal	70-130
After Meal (1-2hrs)	less than 180
Before Exercise	if taking insulin, at least 100
Bedtime	100-140

Amounts shown above mg/dL

A1c	less than or around 7.0%

These are general medical guidelines. Please follow your doctor's instructions.

WebMD

Figure 9.3 Blood Sugar Levels for Diabetics[16]

---

[16] Sources © 2020 WebMD, LLC. All rights reserved.

The CGM

Let me start with the description of devices that are well articulated in the Pocket Guide: *The Continuous Glucose Monitoring, Pocket* Guide is an Endocrine Society and Hormone Health Network Publication. (endocrine.org and hormone.org.)

Pocket Guide

"A blood glucose monitor. Blood Glucose Monitors (BGM), using a test strip measure the amount of glucose in a drop of blood, in a single moment in time, usually taken from a finger. This process is commonly known as a fingerstick. Finger sticks may need to be done several times a day. The results show whether blood glucose is in range at the time performed. This glucose value is often used to make decisions about modifying diet, activity, insulin, or the dosages of other medications…The BGM data can be uploaded to a computer…

…Continuous Glucose Monitoring Systems (CGM) is a newer way for people with diabetes to continuously measure glucose any time. Most CGMs do this by self-insertion of a tiny sensor that you wear for up to 14 days. They come with an easy-to-use inserter, and the sensors have built-in adhesive to help them stick to your skin. Some CGMs last longer but require the sensor to be placed under the skin by a trained professional. CGMs require little to no finger-sticks but do require you to have the receiver/reader or a smartphone nearby. CGMs reports provide detailed insights on trends for day-to-day decisions and for discussions with your provider. CGMs can also automatically collect and share glucose data with a person of your choice and can predict dangerous highs and lows before they happen to help you stay on target."

My Approach

I used to have BGM method of finger sticking with a BGM monitor. It worked well for me until my endocrinologist suggested that I start using a CGM. I still have my BGM as a backup available in case of an emergency.

There are a few CGM systems offered in the marketplace. I have the FreeStyle Libre by Abbott Labs. (https://www.libreview.com/). (There is another one called Dexcom, but I don't know anything about it. I can assume that these would be compatible with the technology. There may be others—I have not researched). My CGM has been a game changer in my diabetes/glucose monitoring. There are two parts to it: A sensor which you place on your upper arm. It has a small needle that does not even pinch. It is good for 14 days. The second part is the reader, which scans the data on the sensor, any time and unlimited times a day. The reader is real-time in that it gives you the entire history of your glucose numbers. The data can be downloaded on a computer, which provides various glucose measures such as TIR and other valuable information for me and my endocrinologist. The physician gives a prescription, which is handled by specialized pharmacies, who send the supplies. I can't imagine managing my diabetes without a CGM. They also have an App with its own reader. It can be downloaded on the mobile phone and is handy when I am away from home. In the US, it is covered by Medicare Insurance.

Following is an Abbott Labs educational chart that shows how the FreeStyle Libre shows moment-by-moment (or at the desired frequency of monitoring) changes in the body's blood glucose level. This enables me to plan what I am going to eat and balance my sugar numbers at any time, all day and night. (https://bit.ly/2SDB9aB)

Current reading	What trend arrow means	Potential reading in 30 minutes
110 ↑	Glucose is rising quickly (more than 2 mg/dL per minute)	>170 mg/dL
110 ↗	Glucose is rising (between 1 and 2 mg/dL per minute)	140-170 mg/dL
110 ↘	Glucose is falling (between 1 and 2 mg/dL per minute)	50-80 mg/dL
110 ↓	Glucose is falling quickly (more than 2 mg/dL per minute)	<50 mg/dL

Figure 9.4 CGM Blood Sugar Indicator

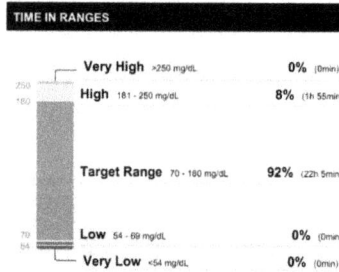

The CGM System provides data that can be downloaded to give a comprehensive view of glucose status—in the desired timeframe. This report, known as the Ambulatory Glucose Profile (AGP) report, allows us to create a more personalized diabetes management plan. The report includes TIR Average Glucose, Glucose Management Indicator, and Glucose Variability. Typically, this AGP report is an especially useful tool when used in conjunction with the A1c number. (Note: Below is my own report as an example.)

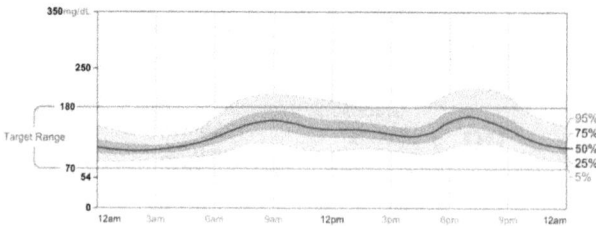

Figure 9.5 CGM AGP Report

Blood Tests

As I was writing this chapter, I had received a note from Quest Diagnostics, the lab I usually go to for my blood tests. Here it is:

"Looking for a smart way to use up your health savings account (HSA) or flexible spending account (FSA) before it expires? Don't let that money go to waste. Check with your health account administrator to see if you can use these funds for QuestDirect™ and choose from nearly 50 lab tests to buy without a doctor visit. Then simply order online, schedule an appointment, or receive an at-home kit, and get results securely through your MyQuest™ account."

These tests include Basic Health Profile, Cholesterol Panel, Complete Blood Count (CBC), Diabetes Management, and Hemoglobin A1c. These are the usual tests my physicians order for me. Normally for these tests, I get a script from my physician, and before my next doctor's visit, I get the test done, which could be every six months or so. While I don't plan to bypass that process, I am pleased to know that I have an option to track my progress on my own—should I want to—more frequently. Of course, there is a cost associated with it, and some States allow these options, and others don't. (New Jersey allows, as I saw on the website). Note there may be other labs with a similar offering.

Shoes for Diabetics

In the US, Medicare medical insurance covers one pair of comfortable shoes per year for diabetics. As diabetes is prone to affect extremities, this is a preventive approach to protect injuries. (I don't know if other insurances cover this). The process is to go through a podiatrist for podiatric care, who determines the need first and then makes an appointment with a pedorthis. The pedorthist is a healthcare professional trained in the science and practice of evaluation and providing therapeutic devices for feet (they contact the physician to verify if one is diabetic and get a formal approval).

Aspirinpod®

It is common knowledge that in case of emergency regarding the feeling of a heart attack and such, one may chew an aspirin (or two) for temporary relief until help arrives. I keep two 325 mg Aspirin pills in a container called Asprinpod, which has a chain attached to it for ease of carrying with car or house keys. Aspirinpod® is a small, sturdy pill container designed to carry an aspirin tablet that could save a life someday. As a gift, I have given these to my family members and friends as well. Last year in the middle of the night, when I felt a feeling of angina, I had chewed two aspirins, and I did get immediate relief until I could dress up and go to the hospital. I consider this to be a first line of defense. <u>As in any other medical-related</u>

considerations, one must consult a physician to get the okay for taking aspirin in such a situation.

Aspirinpod® website https://www.aspirinpod.com/

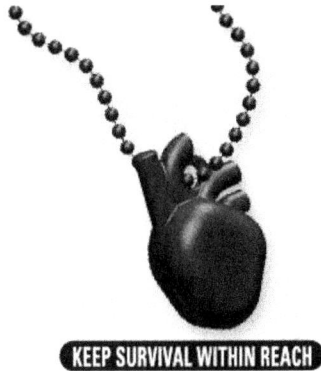

KEEP SURVIVAL WITHIN REACH

Figure 9.6 Aspirinpod®

MedicAlert

I have been a member of the MedicAlert Foundation for many years. I have a tag around my neck-chain which has my identification number and a phone number which, when called, can provide my medical history to the first responders and medical personnel—from anywhere in the world. When I used to travel for business and now for pleasure, I have confidence that should I have an emergency, my medical history will be available immediately. Following is the foundation's website and offering statement.

https://www.medicalert.org/ (Extracted on 1 March 2021)

My Daily Vitals Tracking Template

I diligently maintained a daily log to track my vitals and other important data throughout my initiative of reversing diabetes, healing heart, and weight loss. I had diligently recorded medication intake (particularly inulin doses) and glucose numbers pre- and post-meals. In addition, I had logged the weight and BMI change and general comments about anything that would help understand my body's progress and situation. See Figure 9.7 Vitals Documentation Template.

This became my most important tool to self-observe, self-learn, and adjust my approach on a daily basis. This template was also an effective method for me to discuss my health status with my medical service providers.

Now, after I have been able to eliminate most of the diabetes medication, I have a simplified version of this log—which I continue to maintain daily.

The following spreadsheet log was my tool to manage my health transformation for over one year.

Date	Time	BP	Pulse	O2%	Temp	Insulin BB	Sugar Before Meal /After Meal	Insulin BL	Sugar BM/PK	Insulin BD	Sugar BM/AM	Insulin Long Acting	Total Insulin	Weight
July 14	7a	124/69	75	96		12								181.2
July 17						0	/		/	0	/	22	22	
July 18	6a	127/66	71	98		0	100/130	0	120/150	0	125/140	24	24	179.5
July 20						0	120/150	0	113/135	0	135/205	24	24	
July 21	6a	124/72	70	98	98	0	98/199	0	110/203	0	117/125	22	22	179.2
July 22						0	110/175	0	104/					

Figure 9.7 My Vitals Documentation Template

Maintain a daily hand-written diary. This helps me stay focused on various aspects of my daily routine, which includes my vitals, food, medications, exercises and to-do-list of activities. Rather than type on a computer, I find that old-fashioned-hand-written diary with a fountain pen provides me with a sense of "being in touch" with my plan and actions. And when I check off items, it provides a sense of accomplishment.

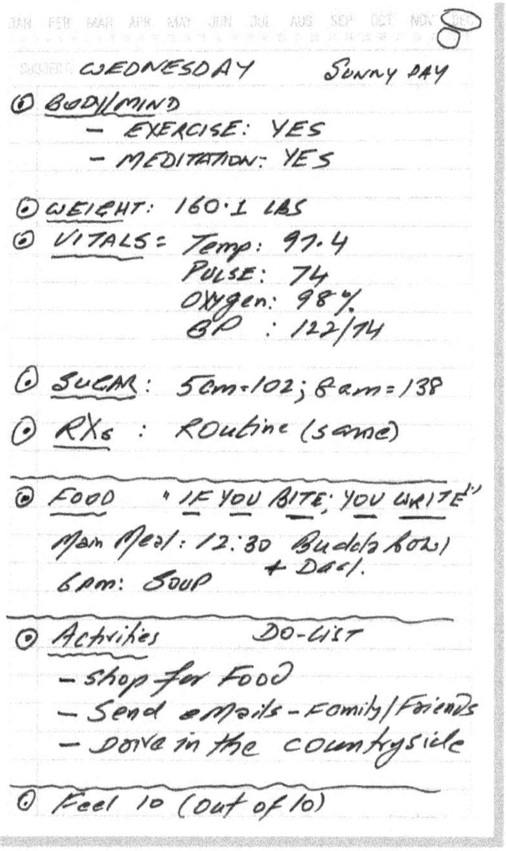
JAN FEB MAR APR MAY JUN JUL AUG SEP OCT NOV DEC 8

SUBJECT: WEDNESDAY SUNNY DAY

⊙ BODY/MIND
- EXERCISE: YES
- MEDITATION: YES

⊙ WEIGHT: 160.1 LBS

⊙ VITALS: Temp: 97.4
PULSE: 74
OXYgen: 98%
BP: 122/74

⊙ SUGAR: 5am=102; 8am=138

⊙ RXs: ROutine (same)

⊙ FOOD "IF YOU BITE; YOU WRITE"
Main Meal: 12:30 Budda Bowl + Daal.
6pm: Soup

⊙ Activities DO-LIST
- shop for Food
- Send eMails - Family/Friends
- Drive in the countryside

⊙ Feel 10 (Out of 10)

Figure 9.8 Daily Diary

After-Action Review

This is a simple yet effective brainstorming tool for assessing any subject or a topic at any given time. The information collected (without judgment) can be useful for making improvements to any initiative. It takes just a few minutes to brainstorm. Business corporations use this methodology for improvement of their products, services, and processes. I find this tool useful to continuously improve my own approach to health and well-being by brainstorming with my family members. Through inclusion in decision-making, this is yet another way of gaining support from your family members.

After-Action Review Template

Date:

Timeframe:

Objective: To gather feedback from spouse/partner/family members for ideas on continuous improvement.

Scope: (define specific purpose of AAR)

I liked (about the topic)	I wish (something to be different)

Table 9.2 After Action Review Template

Below is a real example of a six-month period After-Action Review which I had conducted with my wife to assess her views about my health and wellness transformation. The asterisked (*) items are identified as improvement opportunities.

Date: December 31 Timeframe: July to December.
Scope: My initiative on reversing diabetes, healing heart, and fasting.

I liked (about the topic)	I wish (something to be different)
I am used to it; I am flexible	You could eat more fruit*
You take less insulin and have more control	We could go out to restaurant more often*
Diet used to be good, now it is even better	You have to do what you have to do*
You ask more pointed questions of your physicians, especially the endocrinologist	There were more appealing items to eat on your "Buddha Bowl". *
Loss of weight	
More aware of cooking; and going shopping	
Discovering new things in the store; I would not have even thought of.	
You are researching Insulin Antibody solution	

* After the AAR exercise, the "I Wish" column gave me items that I could improve. I don't eat fruit due to fruticose, but occasionally I started to buy very small-sized apples and tangerines. In the "Buddha Bowl," I have started to add some more nutritious items than before, e.g., *Chyawanprash, Jam with herbs and spices.* When I go out to restaurants (after the pandemic restrictions), I will make a better plan about what I can eat so as not to deny going out with my family and friends.

CHAPTER 10

Conclusion

My last page is always latent in my first; but the intervening windings of the way become clear only as I write.
Edith Wharton (1862-1937), American novelist, short story writer, and designer

A s I reach the end of writing this book, my introspection of thoughts was about the readers. I have documented my health transformation journey as it had unfolded over a period of over one and one-half years giving data to show my before and after health data points.

Before my manuscript goes to the editor and then to the publisher, I wanted to have my latest health data assessed—to prove to myself that I have been able to maintain and sustain my new health profile in these areas of concern: diabetes, the heart, weight, and general well-being. This would be proof that my approach has worked overtime and that I have maintained my discipline, the source of my courage on this transformational journey. I share my latest test data below as proof of sustained continuum after the first major result I shared in Chapter 8

Fasting. There are five areas of my progress outlined in this chapter.

- The Heart
- Bloodwork Profile
- Insulin Autoantibody Analysis
- Genetic Profile for Nutrition & Health
- General Health and Well-being

The Heart (January 2021)

An echocardiogram test was done in my local hospital which showed that my heart is in good condition. While I cannot undo the bypass graft and the stents placed in my heart, I can eliminate and/or minimize the contributing factors causing heart disease.

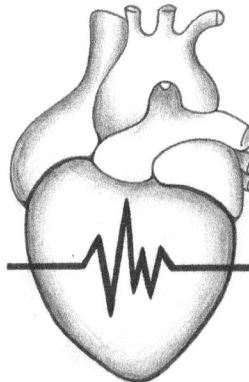

© 2021 ARJIT MAHAL

Figure 10.1 Conceptual Image of Human Heart

Test: The type of study was: *TTE procedure: echo complete 20 doppler 93306.* According to Cleveland Clinic, an echocardiogram (echo) is a graphic outline of the heart's movement. During an echo test, ultrasound (high-frequency sound waves) from a hand-held wand placed on your chest provides pictures of the heart's valves and chambers and helps the sonographer evaluate the pumping action of the heart. Echo is often combined with Doppler ultrasound and color Doppler to evaluate blood flow across the heart's valves. The echocardiogram is performed to test the following aspects of heart-health: Assess the overall function of your heart; Determine the presence of many types of heart disease, such as valve disease, myocardial disease, pericardial disease, infective endocarditis, cardiac masses, and congenital heart disease; follow the progress of valve disease over time; and to evaluate the effectiveness of your medical or surgical treatments. (Reference: https://my.clevelandclinic.org/health/diagnostics/16947-echocardiogram).

The Result. In technical terms for the benefit of the medical professionals, the summary below outlines the positive result as reported by the test result: Normal LV structure and systolic function with apical anteroseptal hypokinesis. LVEF approximately 55-60 %. Normal diastolic function. Normal right ventricle structure and function. No hemodynamically significant valve disease.

No evidence of pulmonary hypertension. No evidence of pericardial effusion.

I am pleased with the result, and so is my cardiologist.

Bloodwork (February 2021)

Except for the Insulin Autoantibody impact. My overall numbers are in range, particularly good and satisfactory — to myself and my physicians. I am on track.

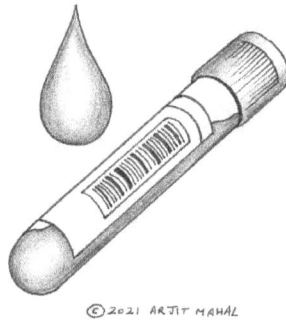

© 2021 ARJIT MAHAL

Figure 10.2 Conceptual Diagram of Blood Test Process

Legend: + Measures are in mg/dL

Measures	Feb 21	+ Measure	Reference Ranges are sourced from Quest Diagnostics' MyQuest Blood Work Report
Lipid Panel, Standard			

Measures	Feb 21	+ Measure	Reference Ranges are sourced from Quest Diagnostics' MyQuest Blood Work Report
Cholesterol, Total	117	mg/dL	Reference Range: <200 mg/dL
HDL Cholesterol	48	Mg/dl	Reference Range: > or = 40 mg/dL *This low number has genetically low. I am told this is genetic! The ration below "matters more!"*
Cholesterol/HDL Ratio	2.4		Reference Range: <5.0 (calc)
LDL Cholesterol	52	Mg/dl	Reference Range: <100 mg/dL This indicator shows that Arteriosclerosis is "not progressing" (CHD) is in better place.
Triglycerides	90	mg/dL	Reference Range: <150 mg/dL
Non-HDL Cholesterol	69	mg/dL	Reference Range: <130 mg/dL (calc)
HS-CRP	1.2		Reference Range: Optimal <1.0 mg/dL Shows Inflammation is "in check".
Hemoglobin A1C	6.3%*		Reference Range: <5.7 % of total Hgb *6.3 is pre-diabetes number.*

Measures	Feb 21	+ Measure	Reference Ranges are sourced from Quest Diagnostics' MyQuest Blood Work Report
C-Peptide	**1.98**	ng/mL	Reference Range: 0.80-3.85 ng/ml
Insulin Autoantibody	**37.5****		Reference Range: <0.4 U/mL. ** This high value shows that my own produced insulin is being attacked and thus making me a type 1.5 diabetic.
Weight in Pounds	**158**		Steady maintenance
BMI	**23.7**		Standard Range: 18.5 – 24.9 Normal or Healthy Weight

Table 10.1 Blood Work & Weight

Insulin Autoantibody Analysis

It was discovered that my pancreas beta cells were not able to produce the required insulin due to damage by the Insulin Autoantibodies' "friendly fire". The beta cells among other type of cells, reside in the pancreas and perform various biological functions. For example, the beta cells secrete insulin while the alpha cells produce glucagon. See Figure 10.3 Conceptual Diagram of Pancreatic Islet.

My doctor had changed my classification from type 2 to type 1.5 diabetes (LADA). In a way, I may be classified as having double diabetes: on the one hand, there is insulin resistance making me a type 2 diabetic, and then insulin deficiency making is making me a type 1.5. diabetic. My physician told me that nothing more could be done regarding insulin autoantibodies because any medication prescribed could harm the overall immune system.

End of the story.

Not that fast. I don't give up that easily. I said to myself: I have an "enemy within"! And I must fight it—somehow.

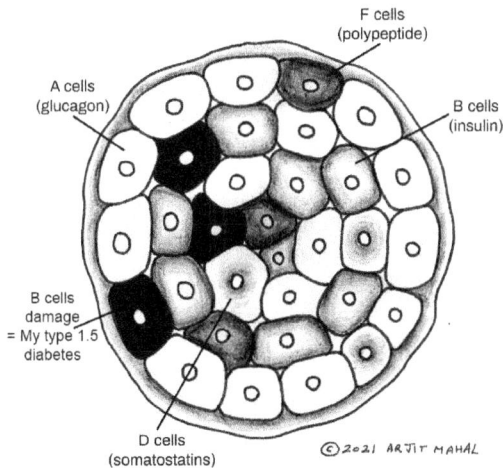

Figure 10.3 Conceptual Diagram of Pancreatic Islet

I decided to see my 95-year-old naturopath physician Dr. Francis J. Cinelli Jr., who always comes up with ideas around issues of health and healing. Before I could say anything, the good doctor said to me, "Artie, I have just finished reading a 400-page book on immune system issues and therapies. It is a complicated subject…I read the book four times before I could make sense of it." "Doc," I said, "you can't see then how could you read the book"? The doctor has failing eyesight due to some problem. He has a gadget that hooks to his eyeglasses and reads the book to him. At his age, some people don't even by green bananas out of concern that they may not live to enjoy them mature for eating. And here, my good friend is seeing patients at this age and researching solutions for his patients. He is truly living the Hippocratic Oath. He is my physician hero! When I told him that I came to see him for advice on my insulin autoimmune problem, he was pleased to get his first test case. His nurse Mary Stein took my blood sample, made plasma out of churning it and off it went to Cyrex Laboratories in Arizona. (https://www.joincyrex.com/the-cyrex-system).

The Test. The test ordered for me was: *Array 6 - Diabetes Autoimmune Reactivity Screen*™. On Cyrex website, it is explained thus: "Assesses markers of the autoimmune components of diabetes. Can be used as a tool to identify reactivity prior to the onset of diabetes and to monitor a patient who is already diagnosed with diabetes to see how well treatment protocols are working. Recommended for Patients Who Have type 1 Diabetes or severe/atypical manifestations of type 2 Diabetes; Have a family history of type 1 Diabetes or Metabolic Syndrome; Have Gluten-Reactivity, Dairy-Sensitivity and/or Cerebellar Ataxia Antigens Tested (IgG + IgA Combined); Glutamic Acid Decarboxylase 65 (GAD65); Insulin + Islet Cell Antigen.

To me, this is all mumbo-jumbo jargon, and I am not about to sign up for a Ph.D. in science. (In humor, the Ph.Ds are sometimes the butt of jokes but let us thank them, they provide a noble service as well).

My test result came as follows:

Array 6 – Diabetes Autoimmune Reactivity Screen

Test	In Range (Normal)	Equivocal	Out of Range	Reference (ELISA Index)
Insulin + Islet Cell		1.67		0.5-1.9
Glumatic Acid Decarfboxylase 65				0.4-1.9

Table 10.2 Diabetes Autoimmune Reactivity Screen Result

Total Serum IgG/IgA/IgM (Total Immunoglobulin Test)

Test Total Serum IgG/IgA/IgM	Low	In Range	High	Reference Mg/dl)
Immunoglobulin G			835.00	751.0-1560.0
Immunoglobulin A			201.00	82.0-453.0
Immunoglobulin M		31.80		46.0-304.0

Table 10.3 Total Immunoglobulin Test Result

The American Diabetes Association in its Diabetes Journal describes the autoantibodies this way: "Islet Cell Autoantibodies: Autoantibodies are created by the immune system when it fails to distinguish between "self" and "nonself." It is normally trained to recognize and ignore the body's own cells and to not overreact to non-threatening substances in the environment. At the same time, the immune system must be able to create antibodies that target and fight specific foreign substances that do pose a threat. The bad news is, when this highly regulated and efficient system is turned onto self-antigens, target tissue damage ensues." (https://diabetes.diabetesjournals.org/content/54/suppl_2/S52)

I am now on a protocol of natural supplements to help my immune disorder.

Will it work? I don't know.

Am I hopeful? Of course, I am.

Genetic Profile for Nutrition & Health

Nutrgenomix, a Chicago-based research organization, specializes in DNA oriented health advice. Their main theme is to eat according to your genes. On the Nutrigenomix website: nutrigenomix.com.

Per dictiory.com, DNA stands for "deoxyribonucleic acid." DNA is a large, complex molecule that carries and passes down the genetic code that makes up all living organisms…DNA has come to metaphorically refer to "the set of nongenetic traits, qualities, or features that characterize a person or thing. "DNA is found in the nucleus of cells of all living organisms. It is arranged in the shape of a double helix, which resembles a twisted ladder. See Figure 10.4 Conceptual Diagram of a DNA Helix."

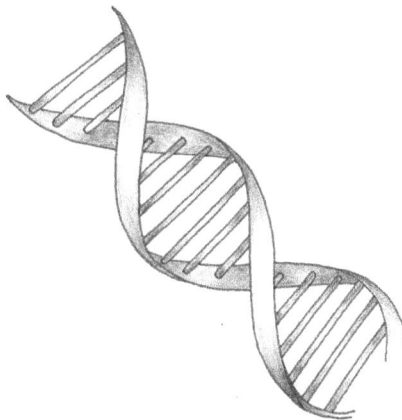

©2021 ARJIT MAHAL

Figure 10.4 Conceptual Image of a DNA Helix

My Personalized Nutrition and Fitness Report

Through a nutritional expert, I had sent my DNA sample to the Nutrigenomix lab, along with details of my diet and other relevant information—as a complete package. After a few weeks, my reports came back. The nutrition expert, who acted as a liaison and a consultant, reviewed the results with me. Following is the outline of the report.

"The Science Behind Nutrigenomix.

One man's food is another man's poison ~ Lucretius.

...The human genome consists of about 25,000 genes, and virtually all can exist in different forms. The variations in our genes make us unique from one another. Genetic variation determines not only the color of our eyes and hair, but how we metabolize and utilize the foods, nutrients, and supplements we ingest.

Nutrigenomics is the science that applies genomic information and advanced technologies to uncover the relationship between genes, nutrition, and human health. The term nutrigenomics refers to both the study of how the food, beverages, and supplements we consume affect our genes and how our genes can influence our body's response to what we consume...understanding your genetic profile and its implications on your unique response to the foods, supplements and beverages you consume will provide you with the tools needed to make the best dietary choices...A healthy, balanced diet should provide enough energy and nutrients to support optimal health, reduce the risk of disease, and maintain healthy body weight."

I found this report comprehensive and a bit overwhelming at first due to the mass of data about my body's elements. However, on closer examination, it started to make sense that the report details are like a mirror from which I can understand and focus on what would matter most to me. For example, the report identifies deficiencies or excesses in considerations like caffeine, sodium, gluten, folic acid, Vitamin B12, and Vitamin D, which greatly affect modifying food habits to improve health. (Not every person needs to be on a salt, caffeine, or gluten restrictive diet.)

The report categories and the associated details include Nutrient Metabolism, Food Intolerance and Sensitivities, Cardiometabolic Health, Weight Management and Body Composition, Eating Habits, Exercise Physiology, and Dietary Recommendations.

I was concerned that I might have to get a Ph.D. to understand the technical jargon. However, I am in the preliminary stage of taking it all in—and it can be overwhelming, but I am confident that based on the data, I can easily understand the basics of what I need to know. As a result, I can adjust my eating habits, lifestyle, and intake of macro and micronutrients such as supplements and vitamins. I would go so far as to say that this information can fill the void for an individual's need when we know most physicians are not knowledgeable in providing advice in micronutrients, as discussed in Chapter 2: Self-Advocacy.

This is still a work in progress for me, and I am looking forward to incorporating the new finding in my health transformation.

General Health and Well-Being

From the origin of life to the progression of its journey in time, complex biological process shapes our destiny. The awareness of "I am" to the spirit within, and then the maintenance of one's body and mind are basic to human existence. See Figure 10.5 Conceptual Image of My Wellness Philosophy.

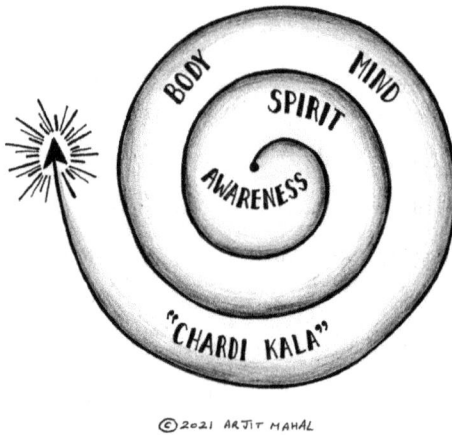

© 2021 ARJIT MAHAL

Figure 10.5 Conceptual Image of My Wellness Philosophy

My goal has been four-fold: Undo Diabetes, Heal Heart, Lose Weight and maintain my general Well-being.

Undo Diabetes: meaning stop, slow the progression of the disorder, and even reverse the potential of damage to the body—to the extent possible. I no longer need insulin four times a day. Now I take it only on ad hoc basis and continue to explore other options.

Heal Heart: while nothing can be done about the bypass grafts and implanted stents in the arteries, there are contributing and damaging factors which can be eliminated or at least minimized to protect further deteriorating condition by managing lipid profile, blood pressure, stress, fitness, and nutrition. Table 10.1 Blood Work & Weight in Chapter 8. Fasting shows the proof that I have been able to achieve and maintain my good numbers over time.

Lose Weight: Thanks to the concept of fasting for autophagy, combined with my self-discipline of food and fitness, I have been able to lose and maintain my weight to the desired number. From 193 pounds at the peak, I am down to 158 pounds with a desirable BMI.

Well-being: This term is complicated because there are many facets of life and living that contribute to one's health and well-being. Broadly, it can include spiritual awareness, body and mind engagement in life's purpose with the spark—the spirit within. I give special credit to my "Chardi Kala".

The term spirit or uplifting of spirit in my mother-tongue Panjabi is referenced as *"Chardi Kala"*; *"Sarbat Da Bhala"*. *"Chardi"* means having an ascending or positive attitude and energy with self-satisfaction and self-dignity in all situations; and *"Kala"* means the art of aspiring to maintain a mental state of eternal optimism and contentment. And *"Sarbat Da Bhala"* is an invocation for the well-being of all humanity—all life—everywhere. These concepts originated from the philosophy of India's Guru Nanak (1469-1539), the first spiritual master, and then continued to be fostered in the psyche of the followers known as the Sikhs by the teachings of subsequent nine masters. By the precepts of Service (*Sewa*), Charity; (*Daan*), and Acceptance (*Bhana*) of the divine will, *"Chardi Kala"* is rooted in all aspects of life and living of the Sikhs.

This psyche of *Chardi Kala* differentiates the Sikh community—no matter where they live in the world, what work they do and what adversities they may face.

With immense gratitude to those who have helped me in my health trial and transformation, and with the privilege of **Chardi Kala**, today I am in a better place.

I invoke from the divine nature, **Sarbat Da Bhala**...well-being of all!

CHAPTER 11

Epilogue

In three words, I can sum up everything I've learned about life: It goes on.

Robert Frost

Recently my wife asked me if I believed in incarnation. I said yes. Now, she had this idea of an Eastern myth that you die and are reborn many times over, go through many lives as animals and insect and such, until you have achieved Nirvana and have earned the right to be born as a human. Then I said, "I don't believe in the mythological belief of incarnation propagated for centuries by the various dogmas; I believe that the incarnation happens in one's lifetime, here and now." When one transforms oneself from a current state of being to another desired state, that is "Nirvana," not the spiritual kind, but simply transformational kind that moves you from current to a desired state, hopefully, a better one. With the present health transformation, I have achieved one form of "Nirvana."

This journey is not a solo venture. I needed support from many aspects. I express my gratitude to all those who helped me, the professionals, book authors, family, and friends. While it may seem that I am naturally disciplined and organized to stick with the programs outlined in this book, it is a daily and diligent effort. There is a big gap between the ideas and actions. Jonathan Wolfgang von Goethe, German writer and statesman, said, "To think is easy. To act is difficult. To act as one thinks is the most difficult."

To motivate myself, therefore, I came up with the principle of: **Courage, Commitment and Compliance.** I remind myself of this personal mantra every day. What nature and life have in store just around the bend of living is not known. I hope to do the best I can, with what I have, till it ends!

The greatest of all time Urdu and Persian poet and philosopher of 19th Century, Asadullah Khan Ghalib, aka Mirza Ghalib, so aptly put it:

"Rau mein hai raksh-e-umar kahaan dekhiye thhamey

Nai haath baag par hai na pa hai rakaab mein."

"Age travels at a galloping pace, who knows where it will stop.

We do not have the reins in our hands, nor our feet in the stirrups."

THE END

References

Internet Addresses given in this book were accurate at the time it went to press.

Books and Periodicals

Austin, Marie. *(2020). Plant Based Diet Cookbook for Beginners.*

Barnard, Neal D. Dr. (2017). *Program for Reversing Diabetes, the Scientifically Proven System for Reversing Diabetes Without Drugs.* RodaleBooks. https://www.rodalewellness.com/.

Castille, Denise. *(2021). I Don't Want To Die Like This: A Survivor's Guide To Thriving After a Heart Attack.* Victorious You Press. https://www.freshstartheart.org/

diaTribeLearn. *Making Sense of Diabetes*: A publication of the diaTribe Foundation, a 501(c)(3) non-profit. Committed to providing free cutting-edge diabetes insights and actionable tips for people with diabetes. https://diatribe.org/

Diet Doctor: *How to Renew Your Body: Fasting and Autophagy,* www.dietdoctor.com

Endocrine Society. *A Pocket Guide to Continuous Glucose Monitoring: Connecting the Dots.* https://www.diabeteseducator.org/docs/default-source/living-with-diabetes/guides/pocket_cgm_guide_english.pdf?sfvrsn=2.

Fung, Jason Dr. *(2016). The Obesity Code, Unlocking the Secrets of Weight* Loss. Greystone Books.

Fung, Jason Dr., & Jimmy More. *(2016). The Complete Guide to Fasting, Heal Your Body Through Intermittent, alternate-Day and Extended Fasting.* Victor Belt Publishing.

Fung, Jason Dr. *(2018). The Diabetes Code Prevent and Reverse Type 2 Diabetes Naturally.* Greystone Books, New York.

Khambata, Cyrus & Barbaro, Robby. (2020). *Mastering Diabetes: The Revolutionary Method to Reverse Insulin Resistance Permanently in Type 1, Type 1.5, Type 2, Prediabetes, and Gestational Diabetes.* Avery, New York. https://www.masteringdiabetes.org/.

Mayo Clinic Foundation for Medical Education and Research publication. (2020). *The Recipe for Healthy Digestion, Steps for Living, Eating and Staying Active.* Product No. 684812. www.MayoClinic.org.

Ornish Living Program Resources: *Ornish Living Newsletter.* https://www.ornish.com/ornish-living/.

Ornish. *Ornish Lifestyle Medicine.* https://www.ornish.com/.

Physicians Committee for Responsible Medicine. (PCRM) https://www.pcrm.org.

Stephens, Gin (2018, September). *Delay, Don't Deny: Living an Intermittent Fasting Lifestyle.*

Organizations & Online Resources

Abbott Labs: *Freestyle Libre*: https://www.libreview.com/

ADCES. Association of Diabetes Care & Education Specialist. https://www.diabeteseducator.org/

American Diabetes Association: https://diabetes.org

Ancient Origins. *Reconstructing The Story of Humanity's Past.* www.ancient-origins.net

Ayur Times. https://www.ayurtimes.com/kala-namak-black-salt-benefits-side-effects/

CDC: https://www.cdc.gov/healthyweight/assessing/bmi/)

Cleveland Clinic Newsroom. https://newsroom.clevelandclinic.org/2017/04/25/cleveland-clinic-researchers-first-show-dietary-choline-gut-bacteria-byproduct-linked-increased-blood-clotting-risk-heart-disease/.

Everyday Health. https://www.everydayhealth.com/

FDA: https://www.fda.gov/food/new-nutrition-facts-label/whats-new-nutrition-facts-label

Game Changers. (2019). Full Movie Documentary. YouTube: https://www.youtube.com/watch?v=ove9b16OeR4

Harvard University: https://www.health.harvard.edu/

Healthline. https://www.healthline.com/

Medic Alert: www.medicalert.org

Medical News Today. https://www.medicalnewstoday.com/

Mindtools. www.mindtools.com

National Heart, Lung & Blood Institute: *BMI Calculation.*

https://www.nhlbi.nih.gov/health/educational/lose_wt/BMI/bmi calc.htm

NIH, National Library of Medicine, National Center of Biological Information. https://pubmed.ncbi.nlm.nih.gov/17510492/

NUTRIGENOMIX: *Eat According to Your Genes. (DNA).* https://nutrigenomix.com/

One Green Planet. www.onegreenplanet.org

The Institute of Functional Medicine. https://www.ifm.org/

University of California: Diabetes Teaching Center at the University of California, San Francisco. *Diabetes Education Online.* https://dtc.ucsf.edu/

University of Sydney Glycemic Index Website. http://glycemicindex.com/index.php

WebMD: https://www.webmd.com/diabetes/mody-lada-diabetes-symptoms-treatment

Yogapedia. www.yogapedia.com

About the Author

Arjit Singh Mahal

Management Consultant, Author, Educator, Historian, and Civic Leader.

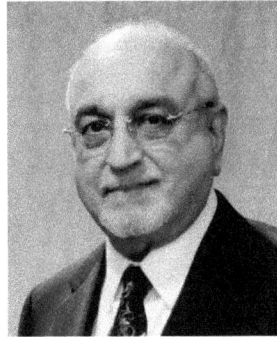

Arjit Mahal had worked as a management consultant and a training manager in a multinational corporation, Mars, Incorporated. He was also the founder of a successful consulting business ASM Group, Inc., and a partner with BPTrends of Boston, an international consulting organization. He had provided professional services on four continents and had been a speaker and trainer at national and international professional forums, which included universities in America and India. (Boston University Corporate Education, Duke University and Chitkara University).

Arjit has been involved in community service most of his adult life. He was the president of the first Sikh Gurdwara (temple) in New Jersey. He had served under three governors of New Jersey as a member of the ethnic advisory council and a member of the historical commission. He has been a member of the Masonic fraternity for over half a century and has served as Right Worshipful Grand Chaplain in the Grand Lodge of New Jersey. He continues to be a member of the Grand Lodge of India.

Arjit lives in New Jersey, USA, with his wife, Millie.

Other books and a documentary by the author:

How Work Gets Done, *Business Process Management, Basics and Beyond.*

Facilitation & Training Toolkit *Engage & Energize Participants for Success in Meetings, Classes, & Workshops.*

After-Action Review, *Continuous Improvement Made Easy.*

Saradrji, *The Man Who Mastered Destiny* (A Biography).

Mahal Gala Village 1952 (Video Documentary on YouTube)

Index

www.ingramcontent.com/pod-product-compliance
Lightning Source LLC
Chambersburg PA
CBHW070916030426
42336CB00014BA/2439